Atlas of Office-based Laryngeal Steroid Injection

Abdul Latif Hamdan

Atlas of Office-based Laryngeal Steroid Injection

Springer

Abdul Latif Hamdan
Department of Otolaryngology – Head and Neck Surgery
American University of Beirut Medical Center
Beirut, Lebanon

ISBN 978-3-032-05234-6 ISBN 978-3-032-05235-3 (eBook)
https://doi.org/10.1007/978-3-032-05235-3

This Springer imprint is published by the registered company Springer Nature Switzerland AG
The registered company address is: Gewerbestrasse 11, 6330 Cham, Switzerland

This book is dedicated to my wife Sawsan for her constant love and support, and to my children, Aya, Adam, and Jad, for being the light of my life.

Preface

Corticosteroid injections are commonly used for the treatment of acute and chronic laryngeal disorders. The main advantage lies in the delivery of a high drug concentration within the lesion while avoiding the risk of adverse systemic effects. The last two decades witnessed a reform in laryngology practice with a shift in laryngeal surgeries from the operating room to the office. This shift has spared the patient the risk of general anesthesia and allowed physicians to treat an array of laryngeal pathologies in an office setting. Patients with various diseases of the upper aerodigestive system can be offered office-based laryngeal procedures such as laser therapy and injections of many pharmaceutical agents among which are steroids.

The *Atlas of Office-Based Laryngeal Steroid Injections* provides an overview of the use of steroids for the management of inflammatory diseases of the larynx in an office setting. More than 100 laryngeal endoscopic images and 10 videos are available to the readers, offering insights on the surgical techniques and outcome of intralesional injections using different approaches. Chapter 1 examines the types of steroids used in laryngology, their indications and dosages, whereas Chap. 2 reviews the different methods for the application of topical anesthesia to the larynx and pharynx. Chapter 3 discusses the approaches used in laryngeal injections, their advantages and limitations. Chapters 4, 5, 6, and 7 review the applications of intralesional steroids injection in the management of exudative lesions of the vocal folds. Endoscopic images of the larynx showing injections of vocal fold nodules, polyps, Reinke's edema, and cysts using the percutaneous and intranasal approaches are presented. Chapter 8 depicts the use of steroids injection as a treatment option for vocal process granuloma, and Chap. 9 explores the added value of intralesional steroid injection following laser therapy for benign lesions of the vocal folds. Chapter 10 presents rare applications of laryngeal steroid injections, and Chaps. 11 and 12 review the use of steroids injection in the treatment of vocal fold scars and laryngeal stenosis. Chapter 13 reviews the rare complications of intralesional steroid injections with emphasis on their self-limiting course.

The author of this book hopes that the *Atlas of Office-Based Laryngeal Steroid Injections* is of use for otolaryngologists who are interested in office-based laryngeal surgeries. The compilation of images and videos represent the author's experience and one perspective in the management of laryngeal disorders using corticosteroids in an office setting.

Beirut, Lebanon

Abdul Latif Hamdan

Acknowledgments

A heartfelt acknowledgment to Dr. Lana Ghzayel for her assistance in reviewing the cases and formatting the manuscript for publication. Her support and dedication were invaluable.

Contents

1 Introduction to Office-Based Laryngeal Injection of Steroids

Corticosteroids are anti-inflammatory medications commonly prescribed for the treatment of inflammatory and autoimmune disorders. They act by inhibiting the release of inflammatory mediators, leading to a decrease in vascular permeability and cellular infiltrates [1–3]. Both long-term and short-term treatment regimens are effective in treating acute and chronic laryngeal inflammatory disorders, thus improving phonatory, swallowing, and airway symptoms. Different synthetic steroids are available on the market, with the most common being prednisone, methylprednisolone, and hydrocortisone (Table 1.1). A major limitation to the use of systemic steroids is their impact on various systems in the body, resulting in an array of undesirable side effects. These include disruptions in glucose and lipid metabolism, osteoporosis, cardiovascular complications, weakened immune function, and delays in wound healing, among many others [4].

Given the adverse effects of systemic steroid use, intralesional injection has been advocated as an alternative. A main advantage of intralesional steroid injection (ILSI) is the ability to deliver a high drug concentration at the site of injection [5, 6]. Numerous studies in the literature support the use of local injections of glucocorticoids in patients with chronic laryngeal inflammatory diseases [7–11]. Hoffman et al. reported ILSI following serial dilatation in 21 patients with granulomatosis polyangitis (GPA) and subglottic stenosis. The use of ILSI obviated the need for tracheotomy in all cases [7]. In a review of 47 patients with GPA and tracheobronchial stenosis, Terrier et al. noted the added value of local steroid injection in reducing failure of endoscopic surgery [8]. Similarly, Krespi et al. highlighted the role of ILSI in managing airway symptoms in patients with laryngeal sarcoidosis [11].

In the last two decades, the management of laryngeal inflammatory disorders has shifted from the operating room to the clinic. Intralesional steroid injections are now performed under local anesthesia with successful results (Table 1.2). In a retrospective study of 24 patients with subglottic and tracheal stenosis, Bertelsen et al. found that in-office ILSI obviated the need for further surgical intervention in 71% of their study group [12]. Pan et al. reported improvement in surgery-free interval in

A. L. Hamdan, *Atlas of Office-based Laryngeal Steroid Injection*,
https://doi.org/10.1007/978-3-032-05235-3_1

Table 1.1 Commonly used systemic corticosteroids

Steroid	Brand name	Type	Dose equivalent (mg)	Biological half-life (hours)	Plasmatic half-life (minutes)
Prednisone	Deltasone	Intermediate	5	8–12	30
Methylprednisolone	Solu-Medrol	Short-to-medium acting	4	12–36	180
Dexamethasone	Decadron	Long-acting	0.75	24–72	100–300
Triamcinolone	Kenalog-40	Intermediate-acting	4	12–36	300
Betamethasone	Celestone	Long-acting	0.5	24–72	100–300
Hydrocortisone	Solu-cortef	Short-acting	20	8–12	90

Table 1.2 Most common steroid types used in office-based laryngeal surgery

Steroid	Brand name	Type	Dosage	Biological half-life (hours)	Plasmatic half-life (minutes)
Triamcinolone Acetonide (40 mg/mL)	Kenalog-40	Intermediate-acting	0.1–0.3 mL (8–12 mg)	12–36	300
Methylprednisolone	Solu-Medrol	Short-to-medium acting	0.1–1.0 mL (40 mg/mL)	12–36	180
Dexamethasone (4 mg/mL)	Decadron	Long-acting	0.1–0.3 cc	24–72	100–300
Betamethasone (6 mg/mL)	Celestone	Long-acting	0.1–0.3 cc	24–72	100–300

13 patients with subglottic stenosis) following office-based corticosteroid injection as adjuvant therapy [13]. Franco et al. reviewed their experience in the management of patients with idiopathic subglottic stenosis treated in-office with repeated steroid injections and noted improvement in peak expiratory flow. This latter was very comparable to that of those treated in the operating room surgically, followed by awake repeated steroid injections [14] (Table 1.3).

The successful use of ILSI in SGS has expanded to include vocal fold scars. Vocal fold scars are characterized by an increase in collagen fibers, fragmented disorganized elastic fibers, and an increase in fibronectin, an adhesion molecule that acts as a scaffold and plays a role in the healing process [17–20]. Mortensen and Woo evaluated the efficacy of office-based steroid injections for vocal fold scars among other laryngeal conditions. The authors reported improvement in voice quality and enhancement of mucosal waves on stroboscopy following treatment [16]. In a study of 25 patients with vocal fold scars treated with a single office-based steroid injection, Young et al. reported significant improvements in the Voice Handicap Index (VHI) score, Glottal Function Index (GFI), auditory perceptual evaluation, and phonation threshold pressure. Stroboscopy also showed

Table 1.3 Intralesional steroid injection for subglottic stenosis

Authors (year)	Title	Steroid used	Steroid type	Dosage	Approach
Franco RA Jr. et al. (2018)	Awake serial intralesional steroid injections without surgery as a novel targeted treatment for idiopathic subglottic stenosis	Triamcinolone acetate 40 mg/mL Dexamethasone 4 mg/mL Methylprednisolone 40 mg/mL Betamethasone 6 mg/mL	Intermediate-acting, long-acting, short-to-medium acting	0.5–2 mL	Transcricothyroid/Transnasal
Bertelsen C et al. (2018)	Serial in-office intralesional steroid injections in airway stenosis	Triamcinolone 40 mg/mL	Intermediate-acting	1–2 mL	Percutaneous
Pan DR et al. (2019)	Office-based corticosteroid injections as adjuvant therapy for subglottic stenosis	Triamcinolone acetonide (40 mg/mL)	Intermediate-acting	3 mL	Percutaneous

improvements in glottic closure and mucosal wave [15]. The improvement in vocal fold malleability can be ascribed to a decrease in fibroblast activity, collagen synthesis, and the turnover of other extracellular matrix constituents [21] (Table 1.4).

There is also growing evidence in the literature supporting the use of steroid injections in patients with benign lesions of the vocal folds [22–27] (Table 1.5). In a systematic review, which included 321 patients with nodules, polyps, cysts, Reinke's edema, and vocal fold scars, Wang et al. reported a significant improvement in all voice outcome measures following intralesional steroid injection (ILSI) [6]. Wu et al. reviewed their experience in 28 professional voice users treated with ILSI for vocal fold polyps and nodules and noted significant disease regression in 82% of the cases. The disease regression was associated with a 7-point drop in the VHI-10 score and improvement in other outcome measures [28]. The results of these reports are not surprising given that inflammation is a common denominator to most exudative lesions of the vocal folds. Zettl et al., in in their study on mouse epithelial cells, suggested that glucocorticoids play an important role in forming and maintaining cell-to-cell tight junctions. The authors showed that synthetic glucocorticoid dexamethasone and insulin resulted in an increase in transepithelial electrical resistance consistent with a decrease in paracellular permeability and the formation of tight intercellular junctions [29].

Table 1.4 Intralesional steroid injection for vocal fold scar

Authors (year)	Title	Steroid used	Steroid type	Dosage	Approach
Mortensen M et al. (2006)	Office steroid injections of the larynx	Methylprednisolone 40 mg/mL	Intermediate-acting	0.1–1.0 mL (40 mg/mL)	Transoral
Young WG et al. (2016)	Voice outcomes following a single office-based steroid injection for a vocal fold scar	Dexamethasone (10 mg/mL)	Long-acting	Not mentioned	Transnasal/Transoral

Table 1.5 Intralesional steroid injection for benign vocal fold lesions

Authors (year)	Title	Steroid used	Steroid type	Dosage	Approach
Tateya I et al. (2003)	Steroid injection for Reinke's edema using fiberoptic laryngeal surgery	Triamcinolone Acetonide (40 mg/mL)	Intermediate-acting	0.2–0.3 mL (8–12 mg)	Transoral
Tateya I et al. (2004)	Steroid injection into vocal nodules using fiberoptic laryngeal surgery under topical anesthesia	Triamcinolone Acetonide (40 mg/mL)	Intermediate-acting	0.2–0.3 mL (8–12 mg)	Transoral
Mortensen M and Woo P (2006)	Office steroid injections of the larynx	Methylprednisolone	Intermediate-acting	0.1–1.0 mL (40 mg/mL)	Transoral
Hsu YB et al. (2009)	Percutaneous corticosteroid injection for vocal fold polyp	Triamcinolone Acetonide (40 mg/mL)	Intermediate-acting	0.1 mL (4 mg)	Percutaneous
Lee SH et al. (2011)	Local steroid injection via the cricothyroid membrane in patients with a vocal nodules	Triamcinolone Acetonide (40 mg/mL)	Intermediate-acting	0.2 mL (8 mg)	Percutaneous
Woo JH et al. (2011)	Efficacy of percutaneous vocal fold injections for benign laryngeal lesions: prospective multicenter study	Triamcinolone acetonide (40 mg/mL)	Intermediate-acting	0.15–0.20 mL	Percutaneous

(continued)

Table 1.5 (continued)

Authors (year)	Title	Steroid used	Steroid type	Dosage	Approach
Wang et al. (2013)	Transnasal endoscopic steroid injection: a practical and effective alternative treatment for benign vocal fold disorders	Dexamethasone (4 mg/mL)	Long-acting	0.1 mL	Transnasal
Wang et al. (2015)	Comprehensive outcome research of intralesional steroid injection on benign vocal fold lesions	1:1 mixture of triamcinolone acetonide (10 mg/mL) dexamethasone sodium phosphate (5 mg/mL)	Long-acting	0.1 mL	Transnasal/Transoral
Hamdan AL et al. (2024)	Office-based steroid injection for benign lesions of the vocal folds: case series and review of the literature	Dexamethasone (8 mg/2 mL)	Long-acting	0.1–0.3 cc	Transnasal, percutaneous, peroral

References

1. Campagnolo AM, Tsuji DH, Sennes LU, Imamura R. Steroid injection in chronic inflammatory vocal fold disorders, literature review. Braz J Otorhinolaryngol. 2008;74(6):926–32.
2. Johnson DW. Croup. Review. BMJ Clin Evid. 2014;2014:0321.
3. West JV. Acute upper airway infections. Br Med Bull. 2002;61(1):215–30.
4. Rice JB, White AG, Scarpati LM, Wan G, Nelson WW. Long-term systemic corticosteroid exposure: a systematic literature review. Clin Ther. 2017;39(11):2216–29.
5. Al-Ali M, Anderson J. The role of steroid injection for vocal folds lesions in professional voice users. J Otolaryngol Head Neck Surg. 2020;49(1):50.
6. Wang CT, Liao LJ, Cheng PW, Lo WC, Lai MS. Intralesional steroid injection for benign vocal fold disorders: a systematic review and meta-analysis. Laryngoscope. 2013;123(1):197–203.
7. Hoffman GS, Thomas-Golbanov CK, Chan J, Akst LM, Eliachar I. Treatment of subglottic stenosis, due to Wegener's granulomatosis, with intralesional corticosteroids and dilation. J Rheumatol. 2003;30(5):1017–21.
8. Terrier B, Dechartres A, Girard C, Jouneau S. Granulomatosis with polyangiitis: endoscopic management of tracheobronchial stenosis: results from a multicentre experience. Multicenter Study Rheumatol (Oxford). 2015;54(10):1852–7. https://doi.org/10.1093/rheumatology/kev129. Epub 2015 May 21.
9. Girard C, Charles P, Terrier B, Bussonne G, Cohen P, Pagnoux C, Cottin V, Cordier J-F, Guillevin L. Tracheobronchial stenoses in granulomatosis with polyangiitis (Wegener's): a report on 26 cases. Medicine (Baltimore). 2015;94(32):e1088.
10. Bower JS, Belen JE, Weg JG, Dantzker DR. Manifestations and treatment of laryngeal sarcoidosis. Am Rev Respir Dis. 1980;122(2):325–32.
11. Krespi YP, Husain S, Mitrani M, Husain S, Meltzer CJ. Treatment of laryngeal sarcoidosis with intralesional steroid injection. Ann Otol Rhinol Laryngol. 1987;96(6):713–5.
12. Bertelsen C, Shoffel-Havakuk H, O'Dell K, Johns MM 3rd, Reder LS. Serial in-office intralesional steroid injections in airway stenosis. JAMA Otolaryngol Head Neck Surg. 2018;144(3):203–10.
13. Pan DR, Rosow DE. Office-based corticosteroid injections as adjuvant therapy for subglottic stenosis. Laryngoscope Investig Otolaryngol. 2019;4(4):414–9.
14. Franco RA Jr, Husain I, Reder L, Paddle P. Awake serial intralesional steroid injections without surgery as a novel targeted treatment for idiopathic subglottic stenosis. Laryngoscope. 2018;128(3):610–7.
15. Young WG, Hoffman MR, Koszewski IJ, Whited CW, Ruel BN, Dailey SH. Voice outcomes following a single office-based steroid injection for vocal fold scar. Otolaryngol Head Neck Surg. 2016;155(5):820–8.
16. Mortensen M, Woo P. Office steroid injections of the larynx. Laryngoscope. 2006;116(10):1735–9.
17. Rousseau B, Hirano S, Chan RW, Welham NV, Thibeault SL, Ford CN, Bless DM. Characterization of chronic vocal fold scarring in a rabbit model. J Voice. 2004;18(1):116–24.
18. Rousseau B, Hirano S, Scheidt TD, Welham NV, Thibeault SL, Chan RW, Bless DM. Characterization of vocal fold scarring in a canine model. Laryngoscope. 2003;113(4):620–7.
19. Tateya T, Tateya I, Sohn JH, Bless DM. Histological study of acute vocal fold injury in a rat model. Ann Otol Rhinol Laryngol. 2006;115(4):285–92.
20. Hirano S, Bless DM, Rousseau B, Welham N, Scheidt T, Ford CN. Fibronectin and adhesion molecules on canine scarred vocal folds. Laryngoscope. 2003;113(6):966–72.
21. Zhou H, Sivasankar M, Kraus DH, Sandulache VC, Amin M, Branski RC. Glucocorticoids regulate extracellular matrix metabolism in human vocal fold fibroblasts. Laryngoscope. 2011;121(9):1915–9.

22. Wang CT, Lai MS, Liao LJ, Lo WC, Cheng PW. Transnasal endoscopic steroid injection: a practical and effective alternative treatment for benign vocal fold disorders. Laryngoscope. 2013;123(6):1464–8.
23. Lee SH, Yeo JO, Choi JI, et al. Local steroid injection via the cricothyroid membrane in patients with a vocal nodule. Arch Otolaryngol Head Neck Surg. 2011;137(10):1011–6.
24. Hsu YB, Lan MC, Chang SY. Percutaneous corticosteroid injection for vocal fold polyp. Arch Otolaryngol Head Neck Surg. 2009;135(8):776–80.
25. Woo JH, Kim DY, Kim JW, Oh EA, Lee SW. Efficacy of percutaneous vocal fold injections for benign laryngeal lesions: prospective multicenter study. Acta Otolaryngol. 2011;131(12):1326–32.
26. Tateya I, Omori K, Kojima H, Hirano S, Kaneko K, Ito J. Steroid injection to vocal nodules using fiberoptic laryngeal surgery under topical anesthesia. Eur Arch Otorrinolaringol. 2004;261(9):489–92.
27. Tateya I, Omori K, Kojima H, et al. Steroid injection for Reinke's edema using fiberoptic laryngeal surgery. Acta Otolaryngol. 2003;123(3):417–20.
28. Wu CH, Lo WC, Liao LJ, Kao YC, Wang CT. Vocal fold steroid injection for benign vocal lesions in professional voice users. J Voice. 2023;37(3):472.e1.
29. Zetti KS, Sjaastad MD, Riskin PM, Ratty G, Machen TE, Firestone GL. Glucocorticoid-induced formation of tight junctions in mouse mammary epithelial cells in vitro. Proc Natl Acad Sci USA. 1992;89(19):9069–73.

2 Application of Topical Anesthesia in Office-Based Laryngeal Surgery

Office-based laryngeal surgery has transformed laryngology practice over the last two decades. The introduction of a flexible endoscope with a working channel and the use of glass fibers for the delivery of lasers allowed a significant number of procedures to be performed in an office setting [1]. This reform in practice has spared the patient the risk of general anesthesia and the morbidity of suspension microlaryngoscopy, and has shortened the recovery period following surgery [2]. In addition, it has improved the time efficiency of physicians and patients and has contained costs, which is a major concern in healthcare expenditure. Various laryngeal procedures are performed in an office setting under local anesthesia. These include laryngeal biopsy, laser therapy, injection laryngoplasty, and injection of botulinum toxin, among other pharmaceutical products [3–5].

The success and completion of office-based laryngeal surgery are contingent on patient tolerance. The latter is linked to several factors, including good application of local anesthesia to the upper airway [5]. Application of local anesthesia to the upper aerodigestive tract was first described in the nineteenth century. Cocaine was used to inhibit the initiation and propagation of action potentials by blocking the membranous voltage-gated sodium channels of neural structures. Since its first description, many synthetic local anesthetics have been introduced. These can be stratified as amides, such as lidocaine and prilocaine, or esters such as tetracaine and benzocaine. The most common mode of administration of local anesthetics is via a solution. The onset of action is rapid, within minutes. Lidocaine 2% is the local anesthetic most frequently used in office-based laryngeal surgery [6].

Supplementary Information The online version contains supplementary material available at https://doi.org/10.1007/978-3-032-05235-3_2.

A. L. Hamdan, *Atlas of Office-based Laryngeal Steroid Injection*,
https://doi.org/10.1007/978-3-032-05235-3_2

2.1 Anesthesia to the Nose

Anesthesia to the nose is usually achieved by spraying the nasal cavity with a solution of local anesthetic or by inserting cotton or gauze pledgets soaked with the anesthetic solution, often mixed with a decongestant such as oxymetazoline 0.05% [7]. The rationale behind using a vasoconstrictor is to provide better hemostasis and to widen the nasal cavity. The most commonly used local anesthetics are lidocaine 2% or 4% and tetracaine 2%. Less commonly used are prilocaine 2%, ropivacaine 2%, and bupivacaine 0.25% [8]. The gauze pledgets are kept in the nasal cavity for 10–15 minutes to achieve the desired anesthetic effect. Other effective methods to anesthetize the nose include the use of an anesthetic gel applied gently to the nasal mucosa or the use of an aerosol. There is no consensus on the most effective mode of application of topical anesthetic to the nose. The choice depends on the physician's preference and patient-related factors such as the nasal anatomy.

2.2 Anesthesia to the Pharynx

Topical anesthesia to the pharynx is usually administered by spraying the oral cavity with lidocaine 2% or 4%. A total of eight to ten sprays may be used, and the patient is instructed to inhale during spraying to facilitate the spread of the anesthetic solution to the hypopharynx and larynx [6]. Other effective methods to anesthetize the pharynx include the use of an anesthetic gel that the patient is asked to swallow or an anesthetic solution to gargle with [9, 10]. Once anesthesia of the pharynx is applied successfully, attention is directed to the larynx.

2.3 Anesthesia to the Larynx

Topical anesthesia of the larynx can be achieved in many ways; one is by applying a cotton (soaked with local anesthetic solution) onto the vocal folds using a sponge holder. The sponge holder is usually introduced orally while the patient is asked to protrude his or her tongue. Another method to achieve anesthesia of the larynx is by dripping the anesthetic solution into the laryngeal inlet using a curved cannula introduced perorally. This can be done blindly or under direct vision using a flexible nasopharyngoscope positioned behind the soft palate for guidance. The surgeon should be diligent when introducing the curved cannula, particularly in patients with a strong gag reflex.

Anesthesia to the larynx can also be achieved by instilling the anesthetic solution via the working channel of an endoscope that is introduced transnasally and positioned above the epiglottis. The anesthetic solution is dripped onto the vocal folds while the patient is asked to sustain a vowel (Video 2.1). This phonatory task, referred to as a laryngeal gargle, allows for good dispersion of the anesthetic solution in the larynx and pharynx. The anesthetic solution may also be instilled via a small catheter that is inserted into the working channel of the endoscope.

A fourth method to anesthetize the larynx is by injecting the anesthetic solution into the subglottic area percutaneously. A 25-gauge needle attached to a syringe is inserted into the cricothyroid membrane and advanced into the subglottis. Once the solution is injected, the needle is immediately withdrawn to avoid any injury due to inadvertent coughing [11] (Video 2.2).

Another effective way to deliver the anesthetic solution to the larynx is by using a nebulizer. This method was first described by *Thawley* in 1987, with the main advantage being the avoidance of laryngeal manipulation [11]. The use of a nebulizer allows for even distribution of the aerosol in the pharynx and larynx. This method is useful in patients with a strong gag reflex and in cases where other anesthesia methods are difficult to achieve. Common examples include patients with a large base of the tongue and those with high fat content in the neck that obscures the cervical anatomy.

A less commonly used method to anesthetize the upper airway in office-based laryngeal surgery is the superior laryngeal nerve block. A 25-gauge needle is inserted between the greater cornu of the hyoid bone and the superior cornu of the thyroid cartilage at the site of entry of the internal branch of the superior laryngeal nerve. The needle should be positioned in the thyrohyoid membrane and should not penetrate the larynx. The superior laryngeal nerve block is reserved for patients who fail the transnasal laryngeal approach or the percutaneous injection technique [4, 12].

The choice of method for anesthesia to the larynx depends on the surgeon's expertise and patient-related factors, such as anatomy and tolerance. The patient should be informed that, following application of the topical anesthetic, he or she may experience difficulty swallowing and excessive salivation. The impaired sensation in the pharynx leads to an increase in swallowing time and a prolongation of the intervals between swallows [13].

Topical anesthesia to the pharynx and larynx can also lead to alterations in upper airway reflexes and resistance, although the motor function of the larynx is preserved. Numerous studies have shown preservation of vocal fold motion following topical anesthesia to the larynx [14].

2.4 Complications of Anesthesia to the Upper Airway in Office-Based Laryngeal Surgery

Complications following the application of topical anesthesia to the upper airway are uncommon. Nevertheless, physicians should be alert to the early symptoms and signs of systemic toxicity following the administration of topical anesthesia to the upper airway.

Physicians should also be aware of the disparities in the absorption and efficacy of different topical anesthetics, which can vary with the mode and site of administration of the anesthetic. Stepwise application of the anesthetic solution helps reduce the summation of plasma levels [15].

The toxic symptoms can be divided into neurologic symptoms, such as tinnitus, headache, and confusion, and cardiovascular symptoms, such as hypotension due to peripheral vasodilation and bradycardia. These symptoms are best treated by administering oxygen, which decreases the risk of acidosis and hypoxia [5].

Another rare complication of topical anesthesia to the upper airway is methemoglobinemia, which occurs secondary to the oxidation of hemoglobin, thus reducing its ability to carry oxygen. Methemoglobinemia is best treated with methylene blue [16–18].

References

1. Zeitels SM. The history and development of phonomicrosurgery. In: Sataloff RT, editor. Professional voice: the science and art of clinical care. 4th ed. San Diego: Plural Publishing; 2017. p. 1347–69.
2. Bredenkamp JK, Abemayor E, Wackym PA, Ward PH. Tonsillectomy under local anesthesia: a safe and effective alternative. Am J Otolaryngol. 1990;11(1):18–22.
3. Jourdy DN, Kacker A. Regional anesthesia for office-based procedures in otorhinolaryngology. Anesthesiol Clin. 2010;28(3):457–68.
4. Wang SX, Simpson CB. Anesthesia for office procedures. Otolaryngol Clin N Am. 2013;46(1):13–9.
5. Woo P. Office-based laryngeal procedures. Otolaryngol Clin N Am. 2006;39(1):111–33.
6. Wellenstein DJ, van der Wal RA, Schutte HW, Honings J, van den Hoogen FJ, Marres HA, Takes RP, van den Broek GB. Topical anesthesia for endoscopic office-based procedures of the upper aerodigestive tract. J Voice. 2019;33(5):732–46.
7. Bourolias C, Gkotsis A, Kontaxakis A, Tsoukarelis P. Lidocaine spray vs tetracaine solution for transnasal fiber-optic laryngoscopy. Am J Otolaryngol. 2010;31(2):114–6.
8. Özkırış M, Aydın R, Gencer ZK, Saydam L. Comparison of topical anesthetic effects of lidocaine, prilocaine, ropivacaine, and bupivacaine in transnasal fiberoptic nasopharyngolaryngoscopy. Am J Rhinol Allergy. 2014;28(3):e141–3.
9. Sohmer B, Bryson GL, Bencze S, Scharf MM. EMLA cream is an effective topical anesthetic for bronchoscopy. Can Respir J. 2004;11(8):587–8. https://doi.org/10.1155/2004/780482. PMID: 15611809.
10. Hamdan AL, Sataloff RT, Hawkshaw MJ. Topical anesthesia in office-based laryngeal surgery. In: Office-based laryngeal surgery. New York: Springer; 2022. p. 123–37.
11. Erickson JC III. Surface anesthesia of the airway and larynx. Int Anesthesiol Clin. 1964;2(3):709–24.
12. Thawley SE. Nebulized anesthesia for the nose, pharynx, larynx, and trachea. Laryngoscope. 1987;97(4):499–500.
13. Chee C, Arshad S, Singh S, Mistry S, Hamdy S. The infuence of chemical gustatory stimuli and oral anaesthesia on healthy human pharyngeal swallowing. Chem Senses. 2005;30(5):393–400.
14. Rubin AD, Shah A, Moyer CA, Johns MM. The effect of topical anesthesia on vocal fold motion. J Voice. 2009;23(1):128–31.
15. Rosenberg PH, Heinonen J, Takasaki M. Lidocaine concentration in blood after topical anaesthesia of the upper respiratory tract. Acta Anaesthesiol Scand. 1980;24(2):125–8.
16. Vessely MB, Zitsch RP III. Topical anesthetic-induced methemoglobinemia: a case report and review of the literature. Otolaryngol Head Neck Surg. 1993;108(6):763–7.
17. Hieger MA, Afeld JL, Cumpston KL, Wills BK. Topical benzocaine and methemoglobinemia. Am J Ther. 2017;24(5):e596–8.
18. Taleb M, Ashraf Z, Valavoor S, Tinkel J. Evaluation and management of acquired methemoglobinemia associated with topical benzocaine use. Am J Cardiovasc Drugs. 2013;13(5):325–30.

Different Approaches and Sites of Injection in Office-Based Laryngeal Steroid Injection

3

The reform in laryngology practice from the operating room to the office has allowed surgeons to perform various laryngeal procedures for the treatment of structural, neurologic, and functional voice disorders. These procedures include injection laryngoplasty, laryngeal biopsy, laser therapy, and laryngeal injection of various pharmaceutical agents, including corticosteroids. The most commonly used approaches in laryngeal steroid injection are the peroral approach, the transnasal approach, and the percutaneous approach. The percutaneous approach can be performed through the thyrohyoid membrane, the cricothyroid membrane, and thyroid cartilage.

3.1 The Peroral Approach

The peroral approach is the oldest and most direct approach to the vocal folds, as it follows an uninterrupted path from the lips to the vocal folds. Since its initial description by Green in 1852 and later by Bruening in 1911, its application in office-based laryngeal surgery has markedly increased [1, 2]. The peroral approach is commonly used for the laryngeal injection of various pharmaceutical agents including hyaluronic acid and calcium hydroxyapatite for patients with glottic insufficiency [3, 4], steroids for patients with vocal fold scar and exudative lesions of the lamina propria [5], cidofovir for patients with laryngeal recurrent respiratory papillomatosis [6], and botulinum toxin for patients with laryngeal movement disorders [7].

The peroral approach for laryngeal injections is easy to learn but requires training to master the technique. After successful application of local anesthetic to the oral cavity, pharynx, and larynx, a curved needle attached to a syringe is introduced into the oral cavity and advanced downward into the larynx. The left hand can be used to stabilize the needle as it is advanced toward the site of injection. Proper visualization of the needle in the hypopharynx can be achieved using a flexible

A. L. Hamdan, *Atlas of Office-based Laryngeal Steroid Injection*,
https://doi.org/10.1007/978-3-032-05235-3_3

endoscope positioned behind the soft palate or via a 70° or 90° telescope—that is introduced perorally. If a flexible endoscope is used, it is preferable to introduce it into the nasal cavity contralateral to the site of the vocal fold to be injected.

The assistant performing the transnasal flexible laryngoscopy should be experienced in navigating with the tip of the endoscope without interfering with the path of the needle, or obstructing the view of the vocal folds during injection. If a telescope is used for visualization, the patient is usually asked to protrude or hold his or her tongue. Once the tip of the needle is visualized, the needle is advanced in a vertical direction caudally toward the vocal folds. The flexible laryngoscope is also advanced—to provide better visualization.

In patients with benign lesions of the vocal folds undergoing intralesional steroid injection, the needle is placed submucosally to allow delivery of the drug into the Reinke's space. A bleb is seen along the entire length of the vocal fold.

The main advantage of the peroral approach is direct visualization of the needle tip. This approach also allows the surgeon to control and gauge the depth of insertion of the needle into the vocal fold. Another advantage is the kinesthetic feedback if a curved cannula is used to palpate the lesion before injection. In patients with impaired or fixed vocal folds, palpating the vocal process also allows the surgeon to assess the mobility of the cricoarytenoid joint.

The main disadvantage of the peroral approach is the risk of inadvertent injury to the mucosa of the oral cavity, pharynx, and larynx—which can occur while introducing the curved needle. Another disadvantage is the limited view, particularly in patients with a crowded oropharynx. Common causes of a crowded oropharynx include a large base of tongue, hypertrophic lingual tonsils, and medial bulging of the lateral pharyngeal walls due to excess fat deposition. Another cause that may impair visualization of the vocal folds during a peroral approach is the presence of a retroflexed epiglottis. Last but not least, the peroral approach is difficult to perform in patients with a strong gag reflex. In this case, other approaches for laryngeal injection are recommended.

3.2 The Transnasal Approach

The transnasal approach is a safe and well-tolerated approach for office-based laryngeal surgery. The use of this approach has expanded with the introduction of the flexible endoscope with a working channel—which enabled physicians to introduce flexible "handles," such as needles for the delivery of pharmaceutical agents. The technique of the transnasal approach is familiar to most otolaryngologists who perform diagnostic nasopharyngoscopy in the clinic.

After having administered the local anesthetic to the upper airway, the flexible nasopharyngoscope is gently introduced through the nose to the nasopharynx—and advanced toward the laryngeal inlet until the vocal folds are visualized. Once the tip of the endoscope is positioned above the vocal folds, a flexible needle (25-gauge) attached to a syringe is introduced into the working channel of the endoscope until the tip of the needle is visualized. It is important to engage the needle only when the tip of the catheter has traversed the tip of the endoscope.

In patients undergoing steroid injection for benign lesions of the vocal folds or vocal fold scars, the needle is inserted submucosally—and the drug is delivered into the Reinke's space (Fig. 3.1). In patients undergoing other types of injections, such as hyaluronic acid or calcium hydroxyapatite for vocal fold paresis or paralysis, the needle is inserted posteriorly in the thyroarytenoid muscle lateral to the vocal ligament (Fig. 3.2).

The main advantage of the transnasal approach is the ability to safely bypass the oropharyngeal mucosa by introducing the needle into the working channel of the flexible endoscope. This "non-touch" approach is useful in patients with a strong gag reflex who cannot tolerate the peroral approach.

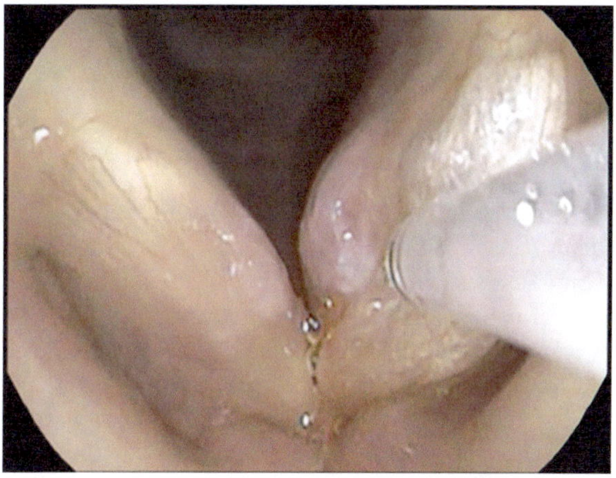

Fig. 3.1 An endoscopic view of the larynx showing an intralesional steroid injection for a left vocal fold fibroedematous mass using the transnasal approach

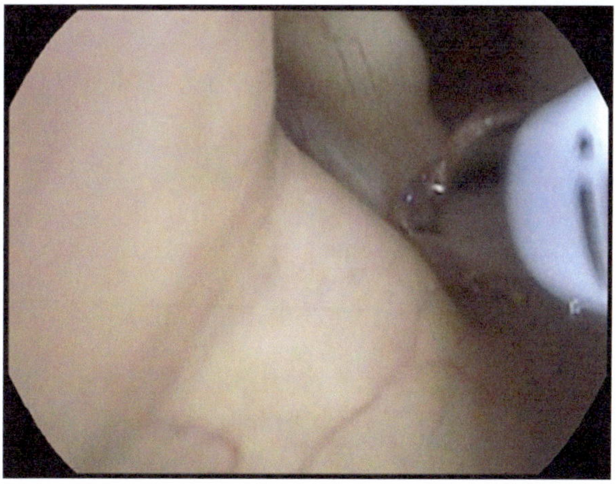

Fig. 3.2 An endoscopic view of the larynx showing a transnasal injection laryngoplasty for a right vocal fold paralysis

On the other hand, the main disadvantage of this approach is the limited visibility and ability to maneuver the needle, as it is coupled to the endoscope. Another disadvantage is the need for a high-pressure device in case the surgeon is injecting a thick substance. It is also important to note the loss of injection material in the dead space of the needle [8, 9].

3.3 The Percutaneous Approach

The percutaneous approach is probably the most common approach used for vocal fold injection. It can be performed via three routes: the thyrohyoid membrane, the cricothyroid membrane, and the thyroid cartilage. All three approaches require proper identification of the laryngeal and cervical landmarks. The skin should be disinfected before inserting the needle, and the application of 2% lidocaine at the site of insertion is optional.

3.3.1 The Thyrohyoid Approach

The thyrohyoid approach was initially described by Getz et al. in 2005 for the treatment of recurrent respiratory papillomatosis (RRP) [10], and later by Amin et al. for the treatment of glottic insufficiency [11]. Despite its popularity among many otolaryngologists, this approach has its limitations [12–14]. Rees et al. reported that 13% of patients undergoing IL in their study group had the procedure aborted due to difficulty with the injection angle [14].

The surgical technique of the thyrohyoid approach is simple. Seating the patient in a "sniff" position helps the surgeon identify the anatomical landmarks of the larynx, mainly the thyrohyoid space and thyroid notch. The tip of the needle should be inserted above the thyroid notch and advanced inferiorly through the preepiglottic space into the laryngeal lumen. A 24–25-gauge needle, 1.5 inches long, is commonly used for the injection of steroids or other pharmaceutical products. In case a more viscous material needs to be injected, a larger needle is recommended. A longer needle is also recommended in patients with large larynges.

Several bent techniques have been described to facilitate access to the anterior one-third of the vocal folds. These include bending the needle near the hub or bending the needle at two sites, referred to as the double-bend technique [11, 15]. Note that the needle should enter the laryngeal lumen at the petiole to facilitate its maneuvering (Fig. 3.3). Clary et al. described the use of a larger needle—an 18-gauge needle—that is inserted into the thyrohyoid membrane and used as an introducer for a smaller gauge needle (25-gauge). This technique facilitates the introduction of a thin needle to the site of injection. It is recommended to insert the smaller needle into the larger one at the start of the procedure and ensure that the tip of the needle does not exceed or pass the tip of the introducer. Once the tip is visualized, the

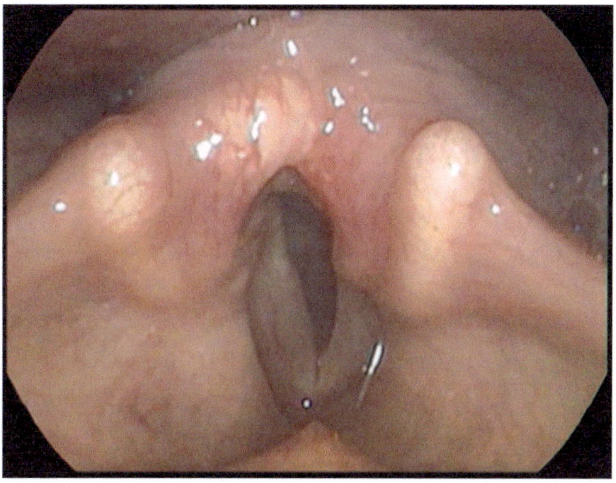

Fig. 3.3 An endoscopic view of the larynx showing a percutaneous injection laryngoplasty for a left vocal fold paralysis

needle is advanced and directed toward the desired site of injection. The tip of the needle can be directed to both vocal folds in patients who need bilateral vocal fold injection.

The main advantage of the thyrohyoid approach is the ability to visualize the needle as it enters the larynx, thus allowing the injection to be performed under vision—unlike the cricothyroid approach, where the injection is performed blindly. However, a main limitation of this approach is the difficulty in identifying the laryngeal anatomic landmarks in obese patients, in those with a history of radiation therapy, or in patients with previous surgery such as a tracheotomy. Another limitation is the difficulty in maneuvering the needle if the entry site in the epiglottis is high or if there is calcification of the thyrohyoid membrane.

3.3.2 The Cricothyroid Approach

The cricothyroid approach was first described by Blitzer et al. in 1988, and has been adopted afterward for the injection of various medications [16]. This approach is easy to perform, with minimal discomfort to the patient. The procedure starts by palpating the cricothyroid space. The pressure exerted externally using an index finger can be seen endoscopically as a bulge between the thyroid cartilage and the cricoid. A 25-gauge needle, 1.5 inches long, is then inserted just above the cricoid cartilage or below the free edge of the thyroid lamina. The entry site can be in the midline or a few millimeters off the midline. The needle can be bent near the hub to help direct the injection toward the desired target. When the needle is inserted in the midline, it passes through the cricothyroid membrane before reaching the thyroarytenoid muscle, where it is directed posteriorly and superiorly. The exact location of the needle can be checked by observing the movement of the vocal fold as you swing the needle vertically or horizontally (Fig. 3.4).

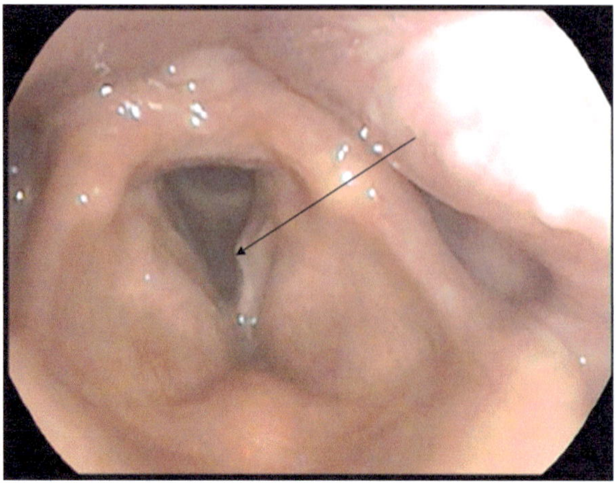

Fig. 3.4 An endoscopic view of the larynx showing the bulge at the site of the tip of the needle that was inserted submucosally via the cricothyroid approach

If the injection is intended to be submucosal, it is important not to violate the laryngeal mucosa. If this happens inadvertently, the patient usually coughs or feels the urge to clear his or her throat. Alternatively, the needle can be inserted 2–3 mm off the midline, usually on the contralateral side where the injection is intended. In this case, the needle penetrates the laryngeal lumen in the subglottic region, thus piercing the mucosal lining. It is then directed superiorly toward the opposite vocal fold where the injection is intended [8, 9, 17].

While performing vocal fold injections using the cricothyroid approach, it is important to note the anatomical variation in the laryngeal structures across genders. In a three-dimensionally reconstructed computerized tomography of the larynges of 14 patients undergoing injection laryngoplasty, Jin et al. noted a difference across genders in the length from the surface of the injection point to the target, and in the angle at the medial surface to reach the target [18]. In a cadaveric study, Mau and Courey also noted a significant difference in the amount of calcium hydroxylapatite needed to medialize the vocal folds in both genders. The authors found that males required 50–60% more injectate than females [19].

The cricothyroid approach is usually well-tolerated by patients. Sulica et al. reported the successful use of the cricothyroid approach in a large percentage of patients undergoing injection laryngoplasty in an awake setting, with no complications noted [20]. Woo et al. reported their experience using the cricothyroid approach in 51 patients undergoing intralesional steroid injection and noted complete or partial remission in 84.4% of cases [12]. Similarly, Hsu et al. reported the completion of ILSI using the cricothyroid approach in 22 out of 24 patients with vocal fold polyps [21].

A main limitation of the cricothyroid approach is the inability to see the tip of the needle as it enters the vocal fold. Another limitation is the difficulty in identifying the anatomical landmarks of the larynx and in introducing the needle, especially in obese patients and those with thick skin.

3.3.3 Transthyroid Cartilage Approach

The transthyroid cartilage approach, also referred to as the transcartilaginous approach, is another percutaneous approach that can be used for laryngeal steroid injection. The needle is usually inserted a few millimeters below a line drawn halfway between the upper and lower edges of the thyroid cartilage. Pressing at this site will allow the surgeon to visualize the passive movement of the vocal folds under nasopharyngeal examination.

Another technique to confirm the correct placement for injection is to insert the needle until it becomes visible submucosally using a flexible laryngoscope. Based on a cadaveric study that included 83 fresh larynges, Cinar et al. noted that the anterior commissure is located at the midline at the junction of the upper two-fifths with the lower three-fifths of the height of the thyroid cartilage in both genders [22].

The main limitation of this approach is the presence of thyroid cartilage calcification. In a radiologic study using computed tomography neck scans of 283 patients, Glikson et al. noted an increase in thyroid cartilage calcification with age in both genders. Moreover, cartilage calcifications were more prominent posteriorly than anteriorly [23]. In another study, which included 359 cephalometric radiographs of healthy adults, Mupaprapu and Vuppalapati reported laryngeal cartilage calcification of various degrees in the third decade and after. Men were more affected than women, and thyroid cartilage calcification was more frequent [24]. Ossification of the thyroid cartilage may prohibit the surgeon from inserting the needle toward the desired site of injection. Moreover, the lumen of the needle may also be plugged by the cartilage matrix, thus hindering adequate control of pressure while injecting the drug.

References

1. Bruening W. Uber eine neue Behanlungsmethode der Rekurrenslahmung. Ver Deutsch Laryng. 1991:18–23.
2. Arnold GE. Vocal rehabilitation of paralytic dysphonia: I. Cartilage injection into a paralyzed vocal cord. Arch Otolaryngol. 1955;62(1):1–17.
3. Dedo HH, Urrea RD, Lawson L. Intracordal injection of Teflon® in the treatment of 135 patients with dysphonia. Ann Otol Rhinol Laryngol. 1973;82(5):661–7.
4. Halderman A, Bryson PC, Benninger M. Safety and length of benefit of restylane for office-based injection medialization. A retrospective review of one institution's experience. J Voice. 2014;28(5):631–5.
5. Tateya I, Omori K, Kojima H, Hirano S, Kaneko KI, Ito J. Steroid injection to vocal nodules using fiberoptic laryngeal surgery under topical anesthesia. Eur Arch Otorhinolarngol. 2004;261(9):489–92.
6. Co J, Woo P. Serial office-based intralesional injection of cidofovir in adult onset recurrent respiratory papillomatosis. Ann Otol Rhinol Laryngol. 2004;113(11):859–62.
7. Ford CN, Bless DM, Lowery JD. Indirect laryngoscopic approach for injection of botulinum toxin in spasmodic dysphonia. Otolaryngol Head Neck Surg. 1990;103(5):752–8.
8. Mallur PS, Rosen CA. Office-based laryngeal injections. Otolaryngol Clin N Am. 2013;46(1):85–100.

9. Hamdan A-L, Sataloff RT, Hawkshaw MJ. Surgical techniques and operative approaches in office-based laryngeal surgery. In: Hamdan A-L, Sataloff RT, Hawkshaw MJ, editors. Office-based laryngeal surgery. London: Compton Publishing; 2022. p. 139–59.
10. Getz AE, Scharf J, Amin MR. Thyrohyoid approach to cidofovir injection: a case study. J Voice. 2005;19(3):501–3.
11. Amin MR. Thyrohyoid approach for vocal fold augmentation. Ann Otol Rhinol Laryngol. 2006;115(9):699–702.
12. Woo JH, Kim DY, Kim JW, Oh EA, Lee SW. Efficacy of percutaneous vocal fold injections for benign laryngeal lesions: prospective multicenter study. Acta Otolaryngol. 2011;131(12):1326–32.
13. Woo SH, Son YI, Lee SH, Park JJ, Pyeong Kim J. Comparative analysis on the efficiency of the injection laryngoplasty technique using calcium hydroxyapatite (CaHA): the thyrohyoid approach versus the cricothyroid approach. J Voice. 2013;27(2):236–41.
14. Rees CJ, Mouadeb DA, Belafsky PC. Thyrohyoid vocal fold augmentation with calcium hydroxyapatite. Otolaryngol Head Neck Surg. 2008;138(6):743–6.
15. Zeitler DM, Amin MR. The thyrohyoid approach to in-office injection augmentation of the vocal fold. Curr Opin Otolaryngol Head Neck Surg. 2007;15(6):412–6.
16. Blitzer A, Brin MF, Fahn S, Lovelace RE. Localized injections of botulinum toxin for the treatment of focal laryngeal dystonia (spastic dysphonia). Laryngoscope. 1988;98(2):193–7.
17. Woo P. Office-based laryngeal procedures. Otolaryngol Clin N Am. 2006;39(1):111–33.
18. Jin SM, Park CY, Lee JK, Ban JH, Lee SH, Lee KC. Transcutaneous injection laryngoplasty through the cricothyroid space in the sitting position: anatomical information and technique. Eur Arch Otolarhinolarngol. 2008;265(3):313–9.
19. Mau T, Courey MS. Influence of gender and injection site on vocal fold augmentation. Otolaryngol Head Neck Surg. 2008;138(2):221–5.
20. Sulica L, Rosen CA, Postma GN, et al. Current practice in injection augmentation of the vocal folds: indications, treatment principles, techniques, and complications. Laryngoscope. 2010;120(2):319–25.
21. Hsu YB, Lan MC, Chang SY. Percutaneous corticosteroid injection for vocal fold polyp. Arch Otolaryngol Head Neck Surg. 2009;135(8):776–80.
22. Cinar U, Yigit O, Vural C, Alkan S, Kayaoglu S, Dadas B. Level of vocal folds as projected on the exterior thyroid cartilage. Laryngoscope. 2003;113(10):1813–6.
23. Glikson E, Sagiv D, Eyal A, Wolf M, Primov-Fever A. The anatomical evolution of the thyroid cartilage from childhood to adulthood: a computed tomography evaluation. Laryngoscope. 2017;127(10):E354–8.
24. Mupparapu M, Vuppalapati A. Ossification of laryngeal cartilages on lateral cephalometric radiographs. Angle Orthod. 2005;75(2):196–201.

4 Office-Based Steroid Injection for Vocal Folds Nodules

Vocal fold nodules are the most common benign lesions of the vocal folds [1]. They are more prevalent in women than in men and may affect all ages [2, 3]. The presenting symptoms include hoarseness, difficulty projecting the voice, and voice fatigue. In professional voice users, complaints such as loss of range, inability to reach the high notes, and volume disturbance are often reported. Acoustic analysis invariably reveals an increase in perturbation parameters—jitter and shimmer—and an increase in noise-to-harmonics ratio (NHR) [4].

On laryngeal examination, vocal fold nodules are bilateral lesions seen at the junction of the anterior and middle one-third of the vocal folds, the point of maximum phonatory stress [5]. Stroboscopy shows normal or minimally impaired mucosal waves, with occasional mucus stasis on the free edge of the vocal folds. The decrease in mucosal waves, when present, is mostly associated with fibrovascular changes in the lamina propria with or without subepithelial scarring. The closure of the vocal folds during phonation is typically described as an hourglass opening [6].

It is important to differentiate vocal fold nodules from physiologic swelling of the vocal folds, often seen in professional voice users following a prolonged performance. Physiologic swellings of the vocal folds are usually translucent, non-fibrotic, and resolve with voice rest [7]. It is also important to differentiate vocal fold nodules from other vocal fold pathologies, such as a cyst on one side and a reactive lesion on the opposite side [8].

On histologic examination, vocal fold nodules are described as acellular lesions limited to Reinke's space. Epithelial membrane thickening is commonly observed. In a histologic study that included 52 vocal fold nodules. Nunes et al. reported basement membrane thickening in 100% of the vocal fold nodules and

Supplementary Information The online version contains supplementary material available at https://doi.org/10.1007/978-3-032-05235-3_4.

A. L. Hamdan, *Atlas of Office-based Laryngeal Steroid Injection*,
https://doi.org/10.1007/978-3-032-05235-3_4

epithelial hyperplasia in 82.14% of the cases. The authors also noted a correlation between these pathologic findings and the clinical diagnosis in 93% of the cases [9].

According to one classification, vocal fold nodules can be edematous, fibro-edematous, or angio-ectatic. Edematous nodules are usually recent in onset and lack epithelial changes, whereas fibro-edematous nodules are more chronic and characterized by acanthosis or parakeratosis of the epithelium and hyaline sclerosis of the lamina propria [10]. Unlike polyps and Reinke's edema, vascular changes are not seen [11]. In an immunohistochemical study of benign lesions of the vocal folds, including nodules, Courey et al. showed an increase in fibronection and collagen type IV, along with thickening of the basement membrane zone [12].

Voice therapy is the first line of treatment for vocal fold nodules. In a survey on the treatment of dysphonia among otolaryngologists, Cohen et al. noted that vocal fold nodules were among the most common three indications for referral to speech-language pathologists [13]. The advancement in technology and the use of telepractice have furthered abidance and adherence to voice therapy over the last decade or so [14]. Voice therapy focuses on improving vocal hygiene and reducing the hyperkinetic phonatory behavior observed in many patients. It includes breathing exercises, lip/tongue trills, and resonant voice techniques among others [15, 16]. The rationale behind these exercises is to restore a new balance in laryngeal tension. Based on numerous studies, the success of voice therapy may reach 90%. Nevertheless, it is important to note that improvement in voice quality is not always accompanied by complete disease regression. In patients who fail voice therapy, surgery is an option.

Microlaryngeal surgery involves creating an incision at the lateral border of the vocal fold nodule and raising a microflap that allows access to the underlying pathology. The lesion is dissected using sharp microscissors and a spatula and removed while preserving the overlying mucosa. At the end of the surgery, a steroid solution may be injected into the surgical bed [17].

With advancements in technology and reform in laryngeal practice toward office-based surgery, intralesional steroid injection (ILSI) under local anesthesia has gained popularity as an alternative to microlaryngeal surgery for the treatment of vocal fold nodules [18, 19]. Wang et al. investigated the effectiveness of ILSI in patients with vocal fold nodules and polyps and reported complete or partial regression in 29 out of 30 patients. The improvement seen on stroboscopic examination was accompanied by a decrease in the Voice Handicap Index 10 (VHI-10) score and an increase in maximum phonation time [20].

Motenson and Woo reported improvement in 82% of singers with vocal fold nodules treated by ILSI. The authors advocated this treatment modality as an alternative to the oral intake of steroids [20]. *Lee* et al. investigated the effect of ILSI via the cricothyroid membrane in 80 patients with vocal fold nodules. The authors reported improvement following treatment in 49% of cases and complete disappearance of the lesion in 44% of cases. Disease regression was associated with significant improvement in the VHI score, acoustic perturbation parameters, and maximum phonation time [21]. In a case series of 81 lesions—including 22 nodules treated with ILSI—*Hamdan* et al. reported complete and partial disease regression in 65% and 35% of the cases, respectively. The disease regression was associated with a drop in the mean VHI-10 score by 7 points [22].

4.1 Case 1

A 32-year-old woman presented to the voice clinic with a history of hoarseness of a few months' duration. The patient denied a history of smoking, allergy, or reflux disease. Her VHI-10 at presentation was 18. Acoustic analysis showed a fundamental frequency (F0) of 199.59 Hz, habitual pitch (HP) of 199.25 Hz, jitter of 1.76, shimmer of 4.02, noise-to-harmonics ratio of 0.12, and voice turbulence index of 0.061. Her maximum phonation time was 7.37 seconds. Flexible laryngoscopy showed bilateral vocal fold fibro-edematous nodules (Fig. 4.1a).

The patient underwent office-based intralesional steroid injection using a 25-gauge flexible needle introduced into the working channel of a flexible nasopharyngoscope (Fig. 4.1b; Video 4.1). A total of 0.1 cc of dexamethasone (8 mg/2 mL) was injected within the lesion. The procedure was tolerated well by the patient, with no complications noted.

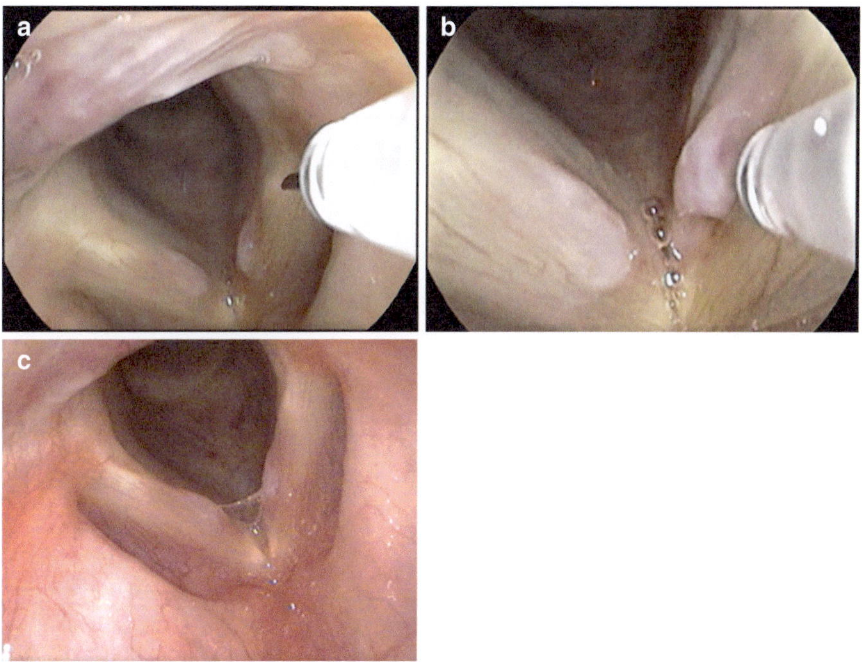

Fig. 4.1 (**a**) An endoscopic view of the larynx showing bilateral vocal fold fibro-edematous lesions. (**b**) An endoscopic view showing the insertion of the needle into the left vocal fold mass. (**c**) An endoscopic view of the larynx 12 weeks following the ILSI showing partial disease regression

On follow-up 3 months later, the patient had partial improvement in her voice quality, with a drop in her VHI-10 score to 8. Acoustic analysis showed an increase in fundamental frequency of 216.29 Hz along with a decrease in jitter of 0.79 and shimmer of 3.78. Laryngeal examination revealed partial regression of the edema on both vocal folds (Fig. 4.1c).

4.2 Case 2

A 52-year-old woman presented to the voice clinic with a change in voice quality. Her Voice Handicap Index-10 (VHI-10) score was 15. Acoustic analysis showed a fundamental frequency (F0) of 196.77 Hz, habitual pitch (HP) of 171 Hz, jitter of 0.72, shimmer of 1.7, noise-to-harmonics ratio (NHR) of 0.07, and a Voice Turbulence Index (VTI) of 0.028. Her maximum phonation time (MPT) was 9.86 seconds. Laryngeal flexible endoscopic examination revealed bilateral nodular swelling, which looked soft and translucent (Fig. 4.2a).

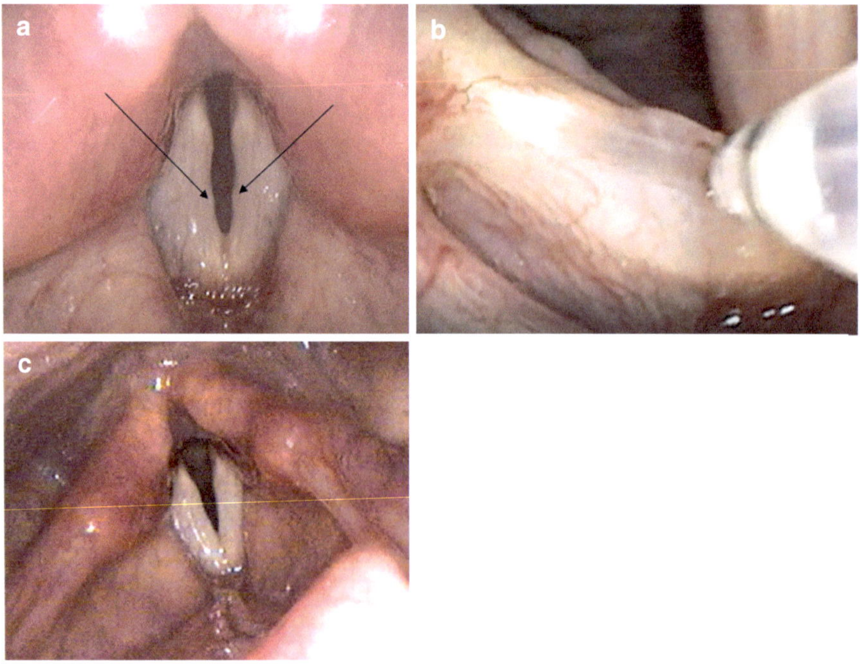

Fig. 4.2 (**a**) An endoscopic view of the larynx showing nodular swelling at the junction of the anterior and middle thirds of the vocal folds. (**b**) An endoscopic view intraoperatively showing the injection of 0.2 cc of dexamethasone (8 mg/2 ml) into the Reinke's space of the right vocal fold. Note the submucosal bulge following the injection. (**c**) Laryngeal examination 6 weeks after the steroid injection showing complete regression of the lesions

The patient was advised voice therapy; however, she elected to undergo office-based steroid injection. The procedure was performed via the transnasal approach using a 25-gauge flexible needle (Fig. 4.2b). A total of 0. 2 cc of dexamethasone (8 mg/2 ml) was injected submucosally into each vocal fold. The procedure was tolerated well by the patient, with no complications noted.

On follow-up 6 weeks later, the patient had a marked improvement in her voice quality. Her VHI-10 score dropped to 7. Acoustic analysis revealed a decrease in the HP to 167 Hz. Laryngeal examination revealed complete regression of the nodules (Fig. 4.2c). The patient was referred to voice therapy to prevent the recurrence of her vocal fold nodules.

4.3 Case 3

A 57-year-old woman presented to the voice clinic with a progressive change in voice quality. The patient had a positive history of voice abuse but denied any history of smoking, allergy or reflux disease. Her Voice Handicap Index-10 (VHI-10) score on presentation was 16. Acoustic analysis showed a fundamental frequency (F0) of 214.05 Hz, habitual pitch (HP) of 228.15 Hz, jitter of 2.52, shimmer of 6.81, noise-to-harmonics ratio (NHR) of 0.21, and a voice-turbulence index (VTI) of 0.071. Her maximum phonation time (MPT) was 8.8 seconds. Laryngeal flexible examination revealed localized edema and mucosal thickening at the junction of the anterior and middle thirds of the vocal folds, suggestive of edematous nodules (Fig. 4.3a).

The patient underwent office-based steroid injection using the transnasal approach. Both vocal fold nodules were injected with a total of 0.3 ml of methylprednisolone (10 mg/1 ml) (Fig. 4.3a–d).

Six weeks following the procedure, she had significant improvement in her voice quality. Her VHI-10 score dropped to 5. Acoustic analysis showed a decrease in jitter of 0.73, in shimmer of 1.71, and in the VTI of 0.009. Her MPT increased to 11 seconds. Laryngeal examination revealed marked regression in the size of the edematous nodules. The patient was advised to undergo voice therapy.

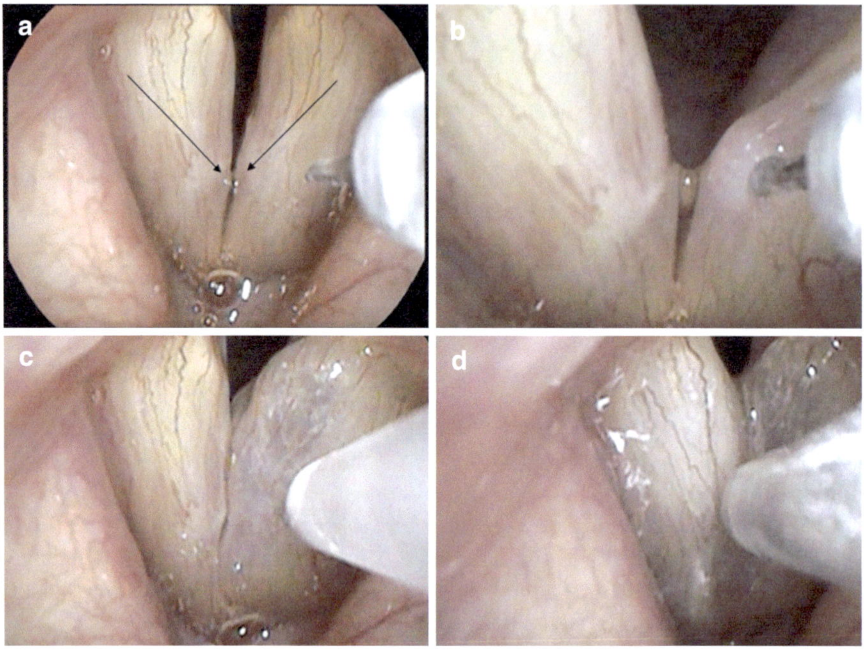

Fig. 4.3 (**a**) An endoscopic view of the larynx showing edema and mucosal thickening at the junction of the anterior and middle thirds of the vocal folds suggestive of early nodules. (**b**) An endoscopic view showing insertion of the needle (25-gauge) into the lesion of the left vocal fold. (**c**) An endoscopic view a few seconds following the injection, showing a bleb formation, which indicates that the injection was made in the superficial layer of the lamina propria. (**d**) A view of the larynx showing the intralesional steroid injection on the right side

4.4 Case 4

A 21-year-old woman presented to the voice clinic with hoarseness of a few months' duration. Her Voice Handicap Index-10 (VHI-10) score was 16. Acoustic analysis showed a fundamental frequency (F0) of 178.85 Hz, habitual pitch (HP) of 166.17 Hz, jitter of 1.09, shimmer of 4.66, noise-to-harmonics ratio (NHR) of 0.115, and a voice turbulence index (VTI) of 0.056. Her maximum phonation time (MPT) was 9.31 seconds. Laryngeal flexible examination revealed localized edema of the vocal folds at the junction of the anterior and middle thirds of the vocal folds, suggestive of vocal fold nodules (Fig. 4.4a). Following voice rest and a short course of steroids, the patient elected to undergo interstitial laser surgery injection (ILSI).

The procedure was performed via the thyrohyoid approach. It was well tolerated by the patient, with no complications noted (Fig. 4.4b, c).

On follow-up 6 weeks later, the patient had significant improvement in her voice quality. Her VHI-10 score dropped to 10. Acoustic analysis showed an increase in

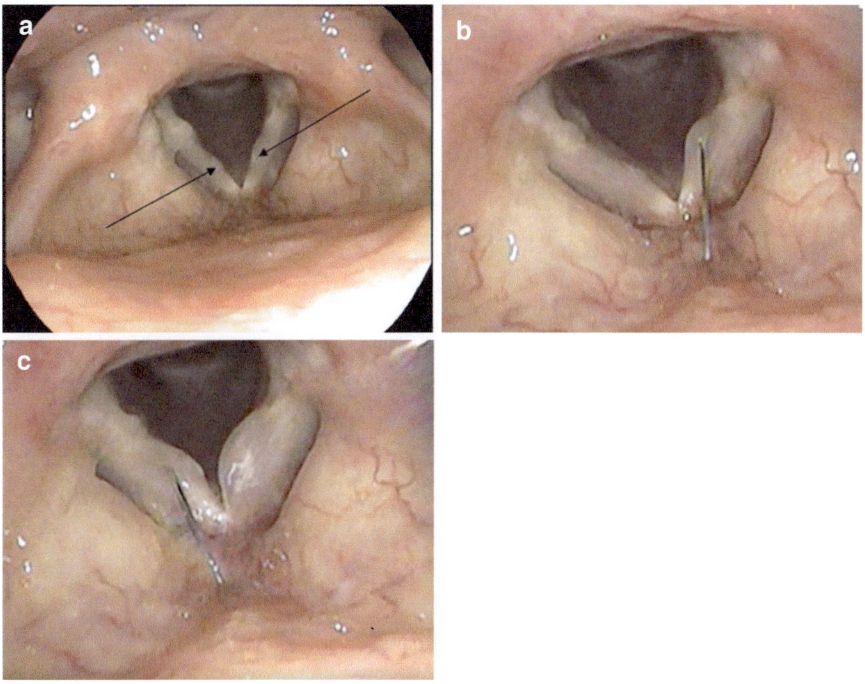

Fig. 4.4 (**a**) An endoscopic view of the larynx showing swelling of the vocal folds at the junction of the anterior and middle thirds of the vocal folds, suggestive of vocal fold nodules. (**b**) An endoscopic view showing the tip of a 25-gauge needle inserted submucosally in the left vocal fold. Note the entry of the needle at the level of the petiole. (**c**) An endoscopic view showing the tip of the needle inserted submucosally in right vocal fold. Note a bleb formation in both vocal folds

the F0 to 206.01 Hz and in HP to 178.34 Hz. There was a decrease in jitter of 0.51 and in shimmer to 2.95. Her MPT increased to 15.3 seconds. Laryngeal examination revealed partial disease regression. The patient was advised to undergo voice therapy and a second office-based steroid injection if needed.

4.5 Case 5

A 22-year-old male patient, a heavy smoker, presented to the voice clinic with hoarseness of a few years' duration. The patient denied any history of allergy or reflux disease. His VHI-10 was 13. Laryngeal flexible endoscopic examination showed bilateral fibroedematous nodules (Fig. 4.5a). The patient underwent office-based steroid injection via the transnasal approach. A total of 0.2 cc of methylprednisolone (10 mg/1 ml) was injected into the fibrovascular nodules using the thyrohyoid approach (Fig. 4.5b). The procedure was tolerated well by the patient, and no complications were noted.

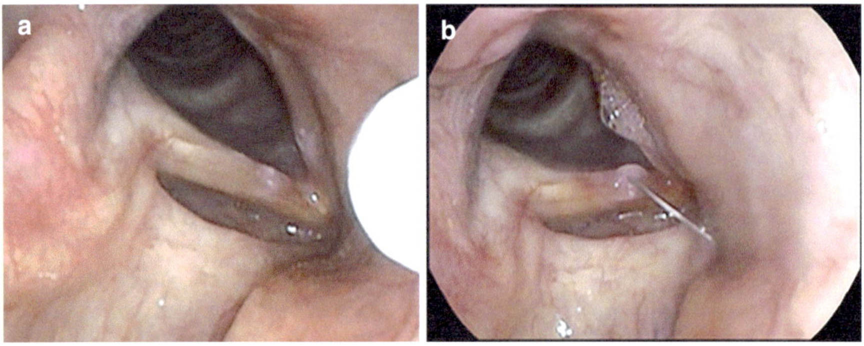

Fig. 4.5 (**a**) An endoscopic view of the larynx showing bilateral fibroedematous masses at the junction of the anterior and middle thirds of the vocal folds. (**b**) An endoscopic view of the larynx showing injection of the right vocal fold nodule using a 25-gauge needle that was introduced via the thyrohyoid membrane

On follow-up a few weeks later, the patient reported mild improvement in his voice quality. Laryngeal examination revealed partial disease regression, for which another injection was performed using the percutaneous thyrohyoid approach.

On his second follow-up, the patient had marked improvement in his voice quality, with a drop in his VHI-10 score to 9. Laryngeal examination revealed further regression of the fibrovascular masses.

4.6 Case 6

A 45-year-old woman presented to the voice clinic with intermittent hoarseness associated with vocal fatigue. The patient denied any history of smoking, allergy, or reflux disease. Her Voice Handicap Index-10 (VHI-10) score was 13. Acoustic analysis showed a fundamental frequency (F0) of 199.33 Hz, habitual pitch (HP) of 179.54 Hz, jitter of 1.7, shimmer of 2.91, noise-to-harmonics ratio (NHR) of 0.125, and a voice turbulence index (VTI) of 0.037. Her maximum phonation time (MPT) was 6.41 seconds. Flexible laryngoscopy revealed bilateral localized edema at the junction of the anterior and middle thirds of the vocal folds suggestive of edematous nodules (Fig. 4.6a).

The patient underwent office-based steroid injection (0.4 cc of dexamethasone 8 mg/2 ml) using a 25-gauge flexible needle introduced into the working channel of a nasopharyngoscope (Fig. 4.6b). The procedure was tolerated well by the patient, with no complications noted.

On follow-up 6 months later, the patient had a significant improvement in her voice quality. Her VHI-10 score dropped to 3. Acoustic analysis showed an increase in the F0 to 208.46 Hz. There was a decrease in jitter of 0.86. Laryngeal examination revealed complete regression of the bilateral lesions (Fig. 4.6c).

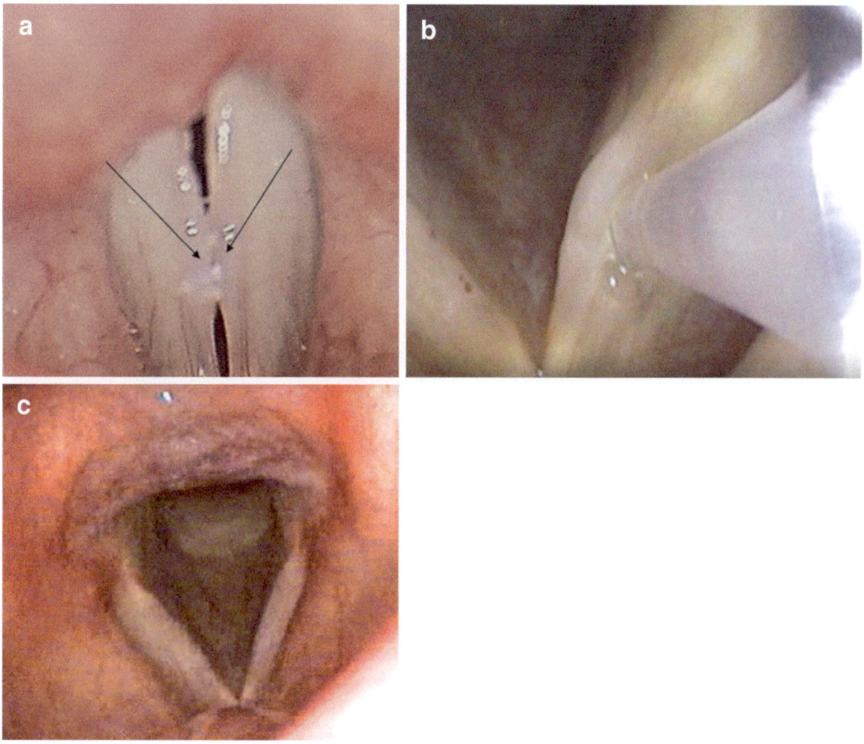

Fig. 4.6 (**a**) A stroboscopic view of the larynx showing an hourglass closure of the vocal folds during phonation at the modal register. (**b**) An endoscopic view of the larynx showing ILSI on the left side. (**c**) An endoscopic view of the vocal folds 6 months after the injection, showing complete regression of the edematous nodules

4.7 Case 7

A 41-year-old woman presented to the voice clinic with hoarseness of a few months' duration. She denied any history of smoking, allergy, or reflux disease. She had a positive history of phonotrauma. Her Voice Handicap Index-10 (VHI-10) score was 11. Acoustic analysis revealed a fundamental frequency (F0) of 178.16 Hz, habitual pitch (HP) of 182.37 Hz, jitter of 0.926, shimmer of 2.25, a noise-to-harmonics ratio (NHR) of 0.140, and a voice turbulence index (VTI) of 0.036. Her maximum phonation time (MPT) was 13.60 seconds. Laryngeal flexible endoscopic examination showed bilateral vocal fold nodules (Fig. 4.7a).

The patient underwent an office-based vocal fold steroid injection under local anesthesia. The procedure was tolerated well by the patient, with no complications noted (Fig. 4.7b, c).

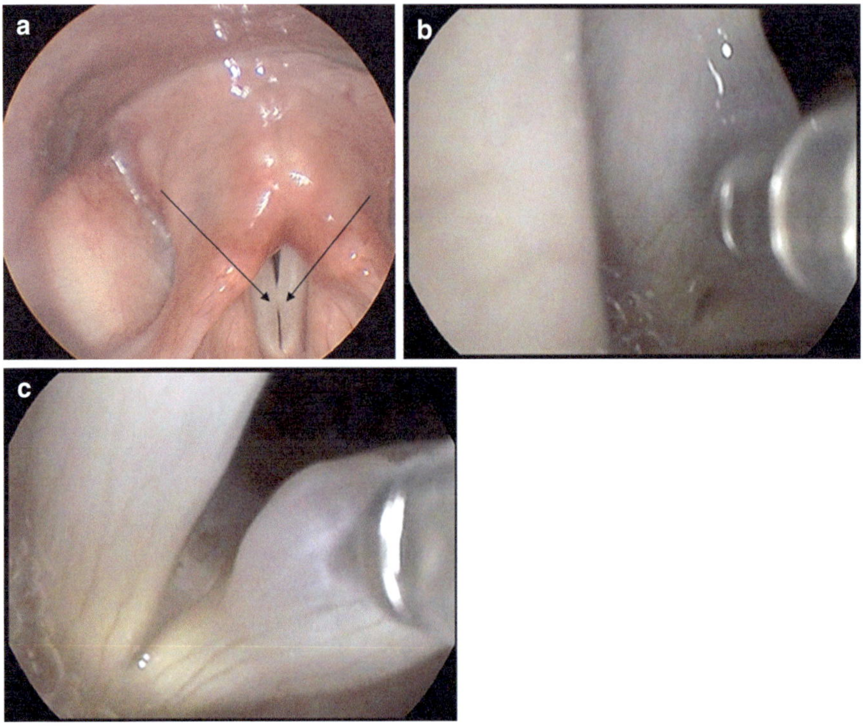

Fig. 4.7 (**a**) An endoscopic view of the larynx showing an hourglass opening of the vocal folds during phonation. (**b**) An endoscopic view of the larynx showing ILSI of right vocal fold nodules. (**c**) An endoscopic view of the larynx showing ILSI of left vocal fold nodules

4.8 Case 8

A 40-year-old woman, heavy smoker, presented to the voice clinic with hoarseness of a few months' duration. The patient had a positive history of voice abuse and denied any history of allergy or reflux disease. Her Voice Handicap Index-10 (VHI-10) score was 18. Acoustic analysis showed a fundamental frequency (F0) of 200.674 Hz, habitual pitch (HP) of 156.75 Hz, jitter of 1.318, shimmer of 2.061, noise-to-harmonics ratio (NHR) of 0.138, and voice turbulence index (VTI) of 0.038. Laryngeal flexible endoscopic evaluation revealed diffuse bilateral vocal fold edema and mild nodular swelling (Fig. 4.8a).

The patient underwent an office-based steroid injection. 0.1 cc of Dexamethasone (8 mg/2 ml) was injected into each vocal fold using the 25-gauge flexible needle (Fig. 4.8b). The procedure was tolerated well by the patient, with no complications noted.

On follow-up 4 weeks later, the patient had mild improvement in her voice quality. She also complained of voice fatigue. Her VHI-10 score dropped to 5. Acoustic analysis revealed a slight increase in the F0 to 202.55 Hz and in HP to 170.07 Hz.

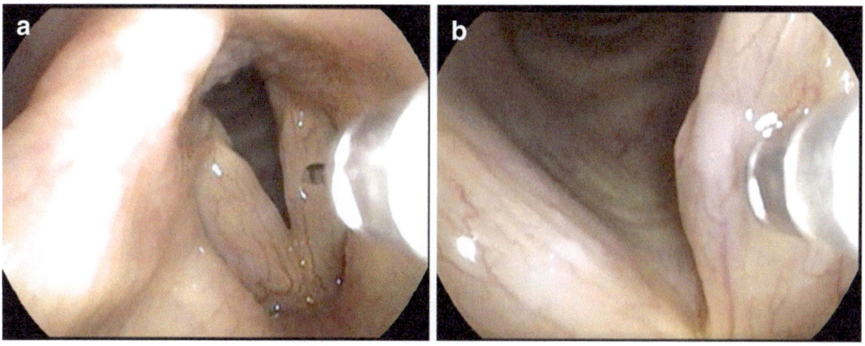

Fig. 4.8 (**a**) An endoscopic view of the larynx showing bilateral diffuse vocal fold edema and mild nodular swelling at the mid-third of the vocal folds. (**b**) Intraoperative view showing left vocal fold steroid injection

There was a decrease in the NHR to 0.114. Laryngeal examination revealed partial regression of the edema on both vocal folds. The patient was advised to cease smoking and undergo voice therapy.

References

1. Woo SH, Kim RB, Choi SH, Lee SW, Won SJ. Prevalence of laryngeal disease in South Korea: data from the Korea National Health and Nutrition Examination Survey from 2008 to 2011. Yonsei Med J. 2014;55(2):499–507.
2. Nagata K, Kurita S, Yasumoto S, Maeda T, Kawasaki H, Hirano M. Vocal fold polyps and nodules. A 10-year review of 1,156 patients. Auris Nasus Larynx. 1983;10 Suppl:S27–35.
3. De Bodt MS, Ketelslagers K, Peeters T, Wuyts FL, Mertens F, Pattyn J, Heylen L, Peeters A, Boudewyns A, Van de Heyning P. Evolution of vocal fold nodules from childhood to adolescence. J Voice. 2007;21(2):151–6.
4. Benninger M, Murry T, Johns MM. Artistic vocal styles and techniques. In: The performer's voice. Plural Publishing; 2016. p. 103–23.
5. Jiang JJ, Diaz CE, Hanson DG. Finite element modeling of vocal fold vibration in normal phonation and hyperfunctional dysphonia: implications for the pathogenesis of vocal nodules. Ann Otol Rhinol Laryngol. 1998;107(7):603–10.
6. Rosen CA, Gartner-Schmidt J, Hathaway B, Simpson CB, Postma GN, Courey M, Sataloff RT. A nomenclature paradigm for benign midmembranous vocal fold lesions. Laryngoscope. 2012;122(6):1335–41.
7. Sataloff R, Hawkshaw M, Sataloff J, Defatta R, Eller R. Idiopathic tracheal stenosis. In: Atlas of laryngoscopy. Plural Publishing; 2013.
8. Niebudek-Bogusz E, Kopczynski B, Strumillo P, Morawska J, Wiktorowicz J, Sliwinska-Kowalska M. Quantitative assessment of videolaryngostroboscopic images in patients with glottic pathologies. Logoped Phoniatr Vocol. 2017;42(2):73–83.
9. Nunes RB, Behlau M, Nunes MB, Paulino JG. Clinical diagnosis and histological analysis of vocal nodules and polyps. Braz J Otorhinolaryngol. 2013;79(4):434–40.
10. Loire R, Bouchayer M, Cornut G, Bastian RW. Pathology of benign vocal fold lesions. Ear Nose Throat J. 1988;67(5):357–8, 360–2.
11. Kotby MN, Nassar AM, Seif EI, Helal EH, Saleh MM. Ultrastructural features of vocal fold nodules and polyps. Acta Otolaryngol. 1988;105(5–6):477–82.

12. Courey MS, Shohet JA, Scott MA, Ossoff RH. Immunohistochemical characterization of benign laryngeal lesions. Ann Otol Rhinol Laryngol. 1996;105(7):525–31.
13. Cohen SM, Pitman MJ, Noordzij JP, Courey M. Management of dysphonic patients by otolaryngologists. Otolaryngol Head Neck Surg. 2012;147(2):289–94.
14. Alegria R, Freitas SV, Manso MC. Is there an improvement on acoustic voice parameters in patients with bilateral vocal fold nodules after voice therapy? A meta-analysis. Eur Arch Otorrinolaringol. 2020;277(8):2163–72.
15. Benninger M, Murry T, Johns MM. Medications: the positive and negative impacts on voice. In: The performer's voice. Plural Publishing; 2016. p. 225–36.
16. Benninger M, Murry T, Johns MM. Complementary and alternative medications and techniques. In: The performer's voice. Plural Publishing; 2016. p. 237–56.
17. Bouchayer M, Cornut G. Microsurgery for benign vocal fold lesions. Ear Nose Throat J. 1988;67:446–64.
18. Wang CT, Lai MS, Hsiao TY. Comprehensive outcome researches of intralesional steroid injection on benign vocal fold lesions. J Voice. 2015;29(5):578–87.
19. Wang CT, Liao LJ, Cheng PW, Lo WC, Lai MS. Intralesional steroid injection for benign vocal fold disorders: a systematic review and meta-analysis. Laryngoscope. 2013;123(1):197–203.
20. Mortensen M, Woo P. Office steroid injections of the larynx. Laryngoscope. 2006;116(10):1735–9.
21. Lee SH, Yeo JO, Choi JI, Jin HJ, Kim JP, Woo SH, Jin SM. Local steroid injection via the cricothyroid membrane in patients with a vocal nodule. Arch Otolaryngol Head Neck Surg. 2011;137(10):1011–6.
22. Hamdan AL, Hosri J, Daou CAZ, Ghzayel L, Hadi J, Saab MB, Kasti M, Mourad M. Office-based steroid injection for benign lesions of the vocal folds: case series and review of the literature. J Voice. 2024:S0892-1997(24)00095-X.

Office-Based Steroid Injection for Vocal Fold Polyps

5

Vocal fold polyps are a common cause of hoarseness in otolaryngology practice. They occur predominantly in men in their fourth and fifth decades, with phonotrauma being the main risk factor [1–3]. In a meta-analysis that included 21 studies, Kwok et al. noted that professional singers were twice as likely to develop vocal fold polyps (OR = 2.1) compared to non-singers [4]. The pathophysiology of vocal fold polyps is multifaceted. One suggested mechanism is an increase in the phonatory stress, which in turn leads to an increase in vocal fold intravascular pressure, bleeding, and high-protein fluid exudation into the lamina propria [5, 6].

Other predisposing factors for the development of vocal fold polyps include smoking and reflux disease. Smoking results in changes in the mucosal lining, such as hyperplasia, metaplasia, or dysplasia. It is important to note that dysplasia is extremely rare and is less frequently encountered in vocal fold polyps compared to Reinke's edema. Smoking also leads to alterations in the constituents of the lamina propria. One example is hyaline degeneration, which distorts the landscape of the Reinke's space [7, 8]. Similarly, reflux disease can cause direct injury to the vocal fold and lamina propria by instigating an inflammatory cascade [9, 10].

Another potential risk factor for vocal fold polyps is *Helicobacter pylori* (HP). In a study on the rate of *H. Pyloric* colonization in larynges of patients with voice disorders, Fang et al. found *H. Pyloric* in 13 out of 33 patients with vocal fold polyps [11].

Patients with vocal fold polyps present with hoarseness, voice fatigue, loss of volume, and repetitive throat clearing. In cases of a large lesion, other symptoms such as dyspnea may prevail. The diagnosis of vocal fold polyps relies on laryngeal examination using a telescope or a flexible nasopharyngoscope. The lesion is usually exophytic and unilateral, seen mostly at the anterior one-third

A. L. Hamdan, *Atlas of Office-based Laryngeal Steroid Injection*,
https://doi.org/10.1007/978-3-032-05235-3_5

of the vocal fold. It can be pedunculated or sessile, gelatinous, or hemorrhagic. A reactive lesion on the contralateral vocal fold may be observed in some cases [12].

In a study of 93 patients with vocal fold polyps who underwent microlaryngeal surgery, Filho et al. noted that two-thirds of the lesions (67.7%) were angiomatous, and one-third (32.3%) were gelatinous. The authors also noted the predominance of angiomatous lesions in men [13]. Narrow band imaging can help assess the vascularity of vocal fold polyps and identify a feeding vessel with a diagnostic accuracy of 96.3% [14]. On stroboscopic examination, patients with vocal fold polyps often exhibit a decrease in mucosal waves and amplitude at the site of the lesion, along with incomplete closure of the vocal folds during phonation [15]. Stroboscopy may also assist in identifying reactive lesions on the contralateral vocal fold or the coexistence of other forms of vocal fold pathology, such as *sulcus vocalis*. Sunter et al. reviewed the medical records of 133 patients with benign lesions of the vocal folds undergoing phonomicrosurgery and noted the presence of *sulcus vocalis* in 49.6% of cases. Their study group included 51 cases of vocal fold polyps, 25 of whom had accompanying *sulcus vocalis* [16].

Histologic examination of vocal fold polyps invariably shows hyaline degeneration, neovascularization, and fibrovascular tissue formation. Mucosal injury, such as atrophy of the epithelial lining and thickening of the basement membrane, may be observed. In a clinicopathologic study of exudative lesions of the Reinke's space, Marcotullio et al. reported abnormal epithelial lining in around 60% of vocal fold polyps [17].

Immunohistochemical staining often shows a change in the direction of the elastin fibers, a decrease in hyaluronic acid concentration, and a significant increase in fibronectin at the basement membrane [18, 19]. Fibronectin is an abundant glycoprotein crucial in regulating multiple functions in the extracellular matrix. The increase in its concentration in vocal fold polyps has been associated with increased vocal fold stiffness [20].

The treatment of vocal fold polyps is surgery, although voice therapy is often advocated as a primary treatment modality. The success of voice therapy in obviating the need for surgery is limited. In a retrospective review of 34 patients with vocal fold polyps, 16 of whom were treated with voice therapy, Klein et al. reported disease regression and improvement in symptoms in 56.3% of the cases [21].

In another review on the effect of voice therapy on disease regression, Nakagawa et al. found that patients with large vocal fold polyps and those with a longstanding history of dysphonia had poorer responses than those with small lesions and short-duration symptoms. The study included 644 participants with vocal fold polyps who had been evaluated before and after treatment [22]. In patients who fail voice therapy, microlaryngeal surgery is recommended. The polyp may be amputated or excised using a medial or lateral mucosal flap [23].

The last two decades have witnessed a reform in laryngology practice. Advances in instrumentation have enabled otolaryngologists to treat vocal fold polyps under local anesthesia. The most accepted in-office treatment modalities are laser therapy and intralesional steroid injection (ILSI). Ramavat et al. compared the outcome of ILSI vs. microlaryngeal surgery in a cohort of 29 patients with small benign lesions, including vocal fold polyps ($n = 19$) who were randomly assigned to one of the two treatment modalities. The authors noted a significant reduction in the size of the lesion following ILSI [24].

In a systematic review of the literature on the role of ILSI for benign vocal fold lesions—including polyps—Wang et al. reported a decrease in the Voice Handicap Index (VHI) score by 27.61 points and an increase in maximum phonation time (MPT) by 1.82 s following treatment. The review included six studies and 321 patients with various vocal fold pathologies [25]. In another study on the recurrence rates following ILSI, Wang et al. noted a failure rate of 24% and 32% at 18 and 24 months following the injection, respectively. In polyps, the long-term effectiveness was noted in almost one out of two patients [26]. Wu et al. investigated the impact of ILSI on voice in 28 professional voice users and found significant disease regression in 82% of the cases, with a drop in the mean VHI-10 score by 7 points (21 preop vs. 14 post-op) [27].

5.1 Case 1

A 32-year-old man presented to the voice clinic with hoarseness of a few months' duration. He had a positive history of smoking, reflux disease, and phonotrauma. He denied any history of allergy. His Voice Handicap Index-10 (VHI-10) score was 13. Acoustic analysis revealed a fundamental frequency (F0) of 113.45 Hz, habitual pitch (HP) of 110.27 Hz, jitter of 0.791, shimmer of 1.522, a noise-to-harmonics ratio (NHR) of 0.131, and a voice turbulence index (VTI) of 0.043. His maximum phonation time (MPT) was 24.12 s. Laryngeal flexible endoscopic examination showed a large polypoid mass on the left vocal fold and a reactive lesion on the opposite vocal fold (Fig. 5.1a).

The patient underwent an office-based intralesional steroid injection. Using a 25-gauge flexible needle, 0.1 cc of dexamethasone (8 mg/2 ml) was injected into the right vocal fold, and 0.2 cc was injected into the left vocal fold (Fig. 5.1b, c). The procedure was well tolerated by the patient, with no complications noted.

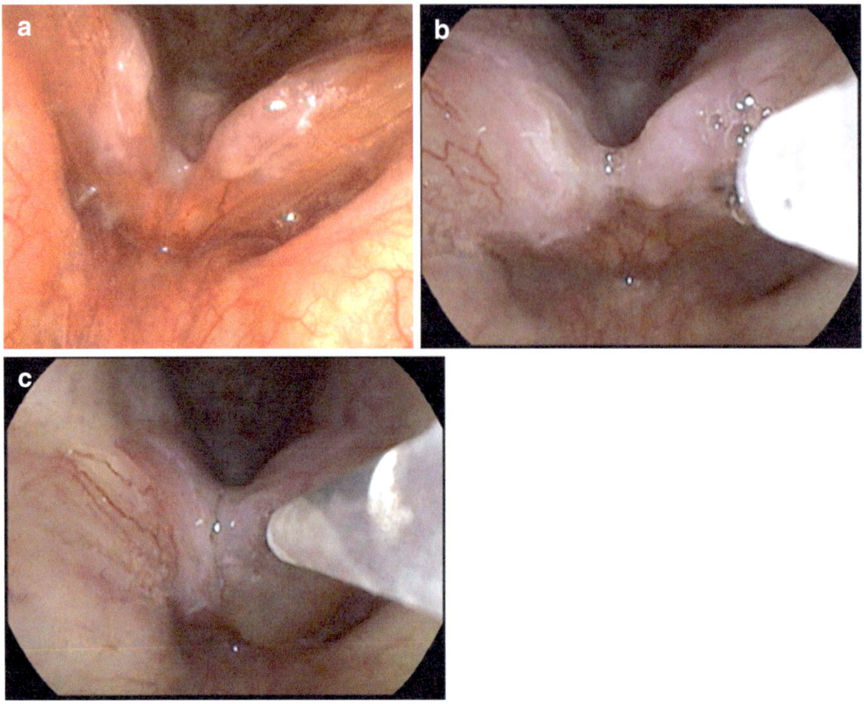

Fig. 5.1 (**a**) An endoscopic view of the larynx showing a left vocal fold polypoid mass, fusiform in shape, occupying almost half of the vocal fold. (**b**) An endoscopic view of the larynx showing insertion of a 25-gauge needle into the left vocal fold polypoid mass. (**c**) An endoscopic view of the larynx showing a bleb formation following the ILSI

5.2 Case 2

A 34-year-old man presented to the voice clinic with a hoarseness of a few months' duration. The patient underwent medical treatment to no avail. He had a positive reflux disease and phonotrauma. He denied any history of smoking or allergy. His Voice Handicap Index-10 (VHI-10) score was 11. Acoustic analysis revealed a fundamental frequency (F0) of 125.8 Hz, habitual pitch (HP) of 125.8 Hz, jitter of 0.549, shimmer of 1.675, a noise-to-harmonics ratio (NHR) of 0.139, and a voice turbulence index (VTI) of 0.054. His maximum phonation time (MPT) was 29.54 s. Laryngeal flexible endoscopic examination showed localized edema of the left vocal fold and a mass formation (Fig. 5.2a, b).

The patient underwent ILSI using the transnasal approach (Fig. 5.2c). A total of 0.2 cc of dexamethasone was injected into the left vocal fold. The procedure was tolerated well.

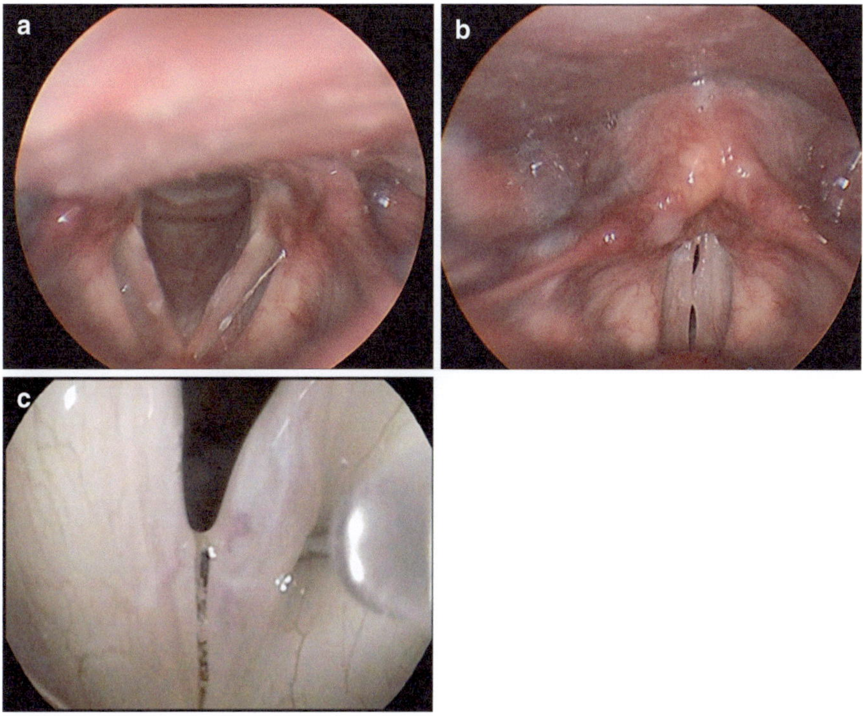

Fig. 5.2 (**a**) An endoscopic view of the larynx showing a left vocal fold localized edema with a fusiform mass formation. Note the mucus on both vocal folds. (**b**) Stroboscopy showing a left vocal fold edema suggestive of an early mass (polyp) during phonation. Note the incomplete closure of the vocal folds. (**c**) An endoscopic view of the larynx showing ILSI into the left vocal fold

5.3 Case 3

A 30-year-old female, a heavy smoker, presented to the clinic with hoarseness of a few years' duration. The patient had a positive history of voice abuse but denied any history of allergy or reflux disease. Her Voice Handicap Index-10 (VHI-10) score was 10. Laryngeal flexible endoscopic examination revealed left vocal fold localized edema.

The patient underwent an office-based steroid injection, and 0.1 ml of dexamethasone (8 mg/2 ml) was injected into the left vocal fold (Fig. 5.3). The procedure was tolerated well by the patient, with no complications noted.

On follow-up 4 weeks later, the patient had marked improvement in her voice quality, with her VHI-10 score dropping to 4. Laryngeal examination showed partial disease regression.

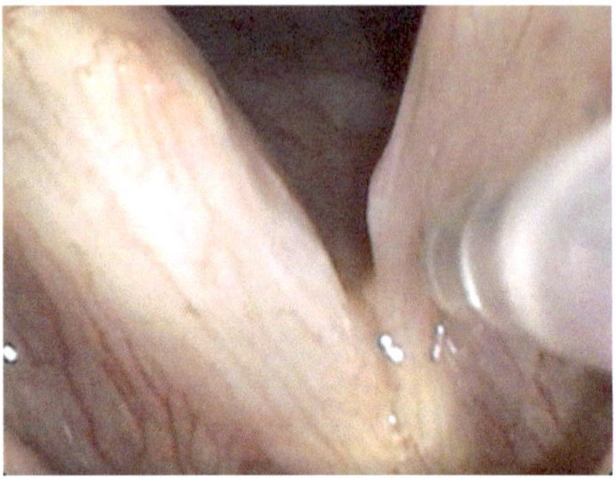

Fig. 5.3 An endoscopic view showing intralesional steroid injection

References

1. Zhukhovitskaya A, Battaglia D, Khosla SM, et al. Gender and age in benign vocal fold lesions. Laryngoscope. 2015;125:191–6.
2. Woo SH, Kim RB, Choi SH, et al. Prevalence of laryngeal disease in South Korea: data from the Korea National Health and Nutrition Examination Survey from 2008 to 2011. Yonsei Med J. 2014;55(02):499–507. https://doi.org/10.3349/ymj.2014.55.2.499.
3. Oliveira P, Ribeiro VV, Constantini AC, et al. Prevalence of work-related voice disorders in voice professionals: systematic review and meta-analysis. J Voice. 2025;39(1):84–104.
4. Kwok M, Eslick GD. The impact of vocal and laryngeal pathologies among professional singers: a meta-analysis. J Voice. 2019;33(1):58–65.
5. Czerwonka L, Jiang JJ, Tao C. Vocal nodules and edema may be due to vibration-induced rises in capillary pressure. Laryngoscope. 2008;118(4):748–52.
6. Titze IR. Mechanical stress in phonation. J Voice. 1994;8(2):99–105.
7. Martins RHG, Defaveri J, Domingues MAC, et al. Vocal polyps: clinical, morphological, and immunohistochemical aspects. J Voice. 2011;25:98–106.
8. Effat KG, Milad M. A comparative histopathological study of vocal fold polyps in smokers versus non-smokers. J Laryngol Otol. 2015;129:484–8.
9. Chung JH, Tae K, Lee YS, et al. The significance of laryngopharyngeal reflux in benign vocal mucosal lesions. Otolaryngol Head Neck Surg. 2009;141:369–73.
10. Lechien JR, Saussez S, Nacci A, et al. Association between laryngopharyngeal reflux and benign vocal folds lesions: a systematic review. Laryngoscope. 2019;129(9):E329–41.
11. Fang TJ, Lee LA, Li HY, et al. Helicobacter pylori colonization in the larynges of patients with hoarseness. Laryngoscope. 2008;118:389–93.
12. Dursun G, Karatayli-Ozgursoy S, Ozgursoy OB, et al. Influence of the macroscopic features of vocal fold polyps on the quality of voice: a retrospective review of 101 cases. Ear Nose Throat J. 2010;89(3):E12–7.
13. Filho JM, Carvalho B, Mizoguchi FM, et al. Characteristics of polypoid lesions in patients undergoing microsurgery of the larynx. Int Arch Otorhinolaryngol. 2013;17(03):279–84.
14. Yılmaz YZ, Uğurlar M, Yılmaz BB, et al. The comparison of narrow band imaging, white light laryngoscopy and videolaryngostroboscopy in the evaluation of benign vocal fold lesions. J Voice. 2023;37:275–81.
15. Rosen CA, Gartner-Schmidt J, Hathaway B, Sataloff RT, et al. A nomenclature paradigm for benign midmembranous vocal fold lesions. Laryngoscope. 2012;122(6):1335–41.

16. Sünter AV, Kırgezen T, Yiğit Ö, Çakır M. The association of sulcus vocalis and benign vocal cord lesions: intraoperative findings. Eur Arch Otorrinolaringol. 2019;276(11):3165–71.
17. Marcotullio D, Magliulo G, Pietrunti S, Suriano M. Exudative laryngeal diseases of Reinke's space: a clinicohistopathological framing. J Otolaryngol. 2002;31(6):376–80.
18. Courey MS, Shohet JA, Scott MA, Ossof RH. Immunohistochemical characterization of benign laryngeal lesions. Ann Otol Rhinol Laryngol. 1995;105:525–31.
19. Cielo CA, Finger LS, Rosa JC, Brancalioni AR. Organic and functional lesions: nodules, polyps and Reinke's edema. Rev CEFAC. 2011;13:735–48.
20. Thibeault SL, Gray SD, Li W, et al. Genotypic and phenotypic expression of vocal fold polyps and Reinke's edema: a preliminary study. Ann Otol Rhinol Laryngol. 2002;111(1):8–14.
21. Klein AM, Lehmann M, Hapner ER, et al. Spontaneous resolution of hemorrhagic polyps of the true vocal fold. J Voice. 2009;23:132–5.
22. Nakagawa H, Miyamoto M, Kusuyama T, Mori Y, Fukuda H. Resolution of vocal fold polyps with conservative treatment. J Voice. 2012;26(3):e107–10.
23. Courey MS, Stone RE, Gardner GM, et al. Endoscopic vocal fold microflap: a three-year experience. Ann Otol Rhinol Laryngol. 1995;104:267–73.
24. Ramavat AS, Tiwana H, Banumathy N, Bakshi J, Panda N, Goel A. Efficacy of intralesional steroid injection in small benign vocal fold lesions. J Voice. 2019;33(5):767–72.
25. Wang CT, Liao LJ, Cheng PW, Lo WC, Lai MS. Intralesional steroid injection for benign vocal fold disorders: a systematic review and meta-analysis. Laryngoscope. 2013;123(1):197–203.
26. Wang CT, Lai MS, Cheng PW. Long-term surveillance following intralesional steroid injection for benign vocal fold lesions. JAMA Otolaryngol Head Neck Surg. 2017;143(6):589–94.
27. Wu CH, Lo WC, Liao LJ, Kao YC, Wang CT. Vocal fold steroid injection for benign vocal lesions in professional voice users. J Voice. 2023;37(3):472.e1–6.

6 Office-Based Steroid Injection for Reinke's Edema

Reinke's edema is a benign disease of the vocal folds commonly encountered in women with a history of smoking. It is characterized by the excess deposition of gelatinous material in the Reinke's space. Other terms frequently used to describe this condition include polypoid corditis, polypoid laryngitis, and polypoid degeneration of the vocal folds [1]. The main etiology of Reinke's edema is smoking. Smoking instigates a change in the lamina propria's extracellular matrix, leading to alterations in its layered structure. Mucosal changes may also occur, ranging from hyperplasia and dysplasia to carcinoma. In a histologic study of 125 patients with bilateral vocal fold Reinke's edema, Marcotullio et al. reported a correlation between the duration of smoking, daily cigarette consumption, and the degree of dysplasia [2].

Another risk factor for the development of Reinke's edema is reflux disease. The retrograde movement of the gastroduodenal contents into the laryngeal inlet results in mucosal edema, hyperemia, and pachydermia. In severe cases, mucosal ulceration and/or granuloma may be seen. In a review on the association between laryngopharyngeal reflux (LPR) and benign lesions of the vocal folds, Lechien et al. noted inflammatory changes and an increase in cell-to-cell dehiscence of the basement membrane [3–4].

Phonotrauma is also a predisposing factor for the development of exudative lesions of the lamina propria. Silva et al. investigated the vocal fold contact pressure in patients with Reinke's edema and found an increase in its amplitude, along with an increase in the phonatory threshold pressure. The study was conducted on two human larynges, and vocal fold oscillations were evaluated using acoustic, aerodynamic, and electrographic measures [5].

The etiologic role of hormonal changes in the development of Reinke's edema has also been investigated. Kravos et al. examined the levels of sex hormones in patients with Reinke's edema ($n = 56$) versus controls with no Reinke's edema. They found a significant difference in testosterone and progesterone between the two groups. The authors concluded that these endogenous hormones affect the

A. L. Hamdan, *Atlas of Office-based Laryngeal Steroid Injection*,
https://doi.org/10.1007/978-3-032-05235-3_6

enzymatic activity of the endothelial wall lining, which, in turn, may contribute to the growth of these lesions [6].

Reinke's edema is characterized histologically by the presence of dilated vessels, plasma exudation, and edematous lakes. Electron microscopic examination shows loosening of the intercellular junctions at the basement membrane and an increase in the intercellular space [7]. In a cross-sectional analysis of 20 specimens of vocal fold Reinke's edema, Sakae et al. reported fragmentation of elastic fibers and disarrangement in the collagen fibers, more so in the deep layers of the lamina propria. The disarrangement correlated with the severity of the disease [8, 9]. Another important finding was the decrease in the concentration of fibronectin, a glycoprotein responsible for strengthening the extracellular matrix of the Reinke's space [10, 11].

The voice characteristics of patients with Reinke's edema are distinctive. Patients present with deepening of the voice, often referred to as "androphonia" in women. In addition to the change in pitch, patients may complain of volume disturbance and difficulty in projecting their voices. Professional voice users can also present with difficulty in sustaining a note and a contracted vocal range. In patients with advanced disease, symptoms such as dyspnea and snoring may prevail secondary to narrowing of the airway. In a study on the pathogenic role of Reinke's edema in obstructive sleep apnea (OSA), Hamdan et al. noted a significantly higher risk of OSA in patients with Reinke's edema in comparison to controls matched by age and gender (36% vs. 4%, respectively) [12].

The diagnosis of Reinke's edema hinges on a proper laryngeal examination. Laryngoscopy shows edema and outpouching of the Reinke's space that extends along the entire length of the membranous portion of the vocal fold. The disease may affect one or both vocal folds to varying degrees. Several grading systems have been suggested based on the severity of the disease. One example is the Tan et al. classification, which stratifies Reinke's edema into four grades. Grade 1 lesions denote 25% narrowing of the airway, whereas grade 4 lesions denote 75% or more obstruction [13]. On stroboscopic examination, there are changes in the mucosal waves as a result of the changes in the viscoelastic properties of the vocal folds [14].

Other findings on stroboscopic examination include asymmetry and aperiodicity, with or without incomplete closure of the vocal folds during phonation. Acoustic analysis invariably reveals a decrease in the fundamental frequency and an increase in the perturbation parameters—jitter and shimmer. Aerodynamic analysis may also reveal an increase in subglottic pressure, with or without an increase in the mean flow rate [15].

The treatment of Reinke's edema is multidimensional. The first line of therapy aims at improving vocal hygiene. Cessation of smoking is crucial for halting disease progression and preventing recurrence. Control of other predisposing factors—particularly reflux disease and phonotrauma—is of paramount importance. In patients who fail voice therapy, surgery may be indicated. Microlaryngeal surgery consists of removing the gelatinous material while preserving the vocal fold mucosal cover. A microflap [16] or mini-microflap [17] is raised to allow exposure to the Reinke's space while averting injury to the vocal ligament. The lesion is dissected submucosally using cold-steel instruments or lasers.

In a review of 14 patients with vocal fold Reinke's edema who were evaluated pre- and post-phonomicrosurgery using "cold-steel" instruments, Schyberg et al. noted disease regression in all cases and an increase in the mean fundamental frequency. The authors also noted that seven of their study group were reoperated because of persistent smoking [18]. The high recurrence rate in patients who smoke should be discussed thoroughly before any intervention. In a study on the long-term effect of surgical treatment of Reinke's edema, Nielsen et al. noted persistent dysphonia in 81% of the cases and recurrence of the disease in 58% of the cases. The study was conducted on 120 patients who had vocal fold stripping and were followed up for 8 years [19].

With the advances in instrumentation, office-based treatment for Reinke's edema has become an acceptable treatment alternative to patients who fail medical treatment and/or refuse to undergo surgery under general anesthesia. In a recent systematic review and meta-analysis that included six studies, Hamdan et al. reported significant improvements in both subjective and objective voice outcome measures following office-based laser therapy. There was a significant decrease in the VHI-10 score associated with significant disease regression. Additionally, there was a significant increase in fundamental frequency and a significant decrease in jitter and shimmer [20]. Another office-based treatment option for Reinke's edema is steroid injection.

A systematic review and meta-analysis that included 321 patients with benign lesions of the vocal folds, Wang et al. showed that intralesional steroid injection (ILSI) resulted in a decrease in the VHI-10 score and in a significant increase in maximum phonation time (MPT). The review included a study by Tateya et al. on 42 patients with Reinke's edema [21]. Takahashi et al. investigated the efficacy of vocal fold steroid injection in 40 patients, 8 of whom were diagnosed with RE, and noted a significant improvement in the VHI score, auditory perceptual rating, and objective voice outcome measures. The authors advocated repeated ILSI as an effective treatment alternative to phonomicrosurgery in patients with RE [22]. Hamdan et al. conducted a retrospective study examining the effect of office-based steroid injection on benign lesions of the vocal folds, including 31 cases of RE. The results showed complete and partial disease regression in 42.9% and 57.1% of the cases, respectively. Disease regression was associated with a significant drop in the VHI-10 score from 17.46 to 6.46 [23].

6.1 Case 1

A 61-year-old woman, a heavy smoker, presented to the voice clinic with hoarseness and voice fatigue. The patient had a positive history of smoking and denied any history of phonotrauma, allergy, or reflux disease. Her Voice Handicap Index-10 (VHI-10) score was 18. Acoustic analysis showed a fundamental frequency (F0) of 144.2 Hz, habitual pitch (HP) of 134.3 Hz, jitter of 1.24, shimmer of 3.3,

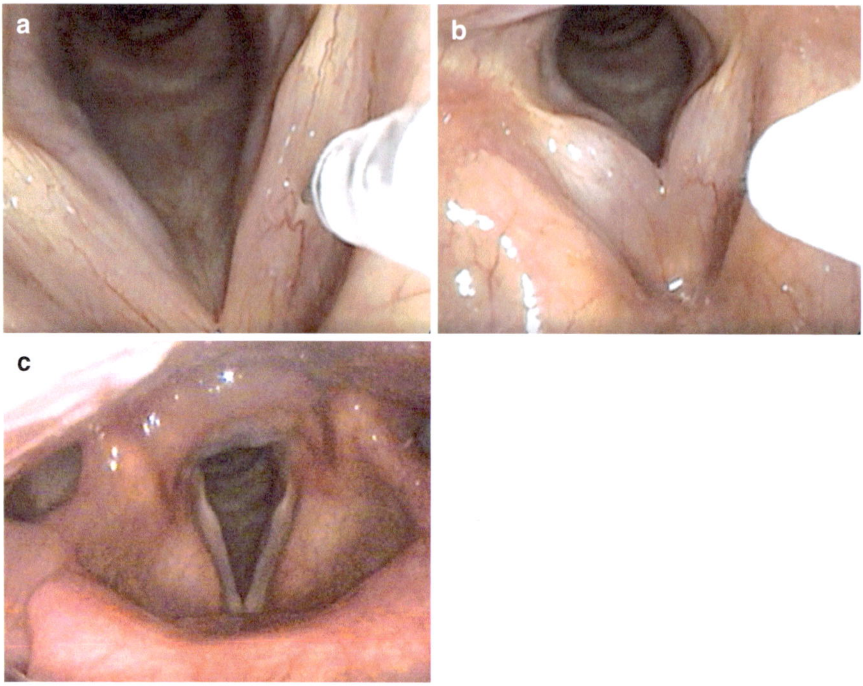

Fig. 6.1 (**a**) An endoscopic view of the larynx showing bilateral type 1 RE. (**b**) An endoscopic view of the larynx following the ILSI. Note the ballooning of the vocal folds. (**c**) An endoscopic view of the larynx 4 weeks after the injection showing almost complete disease regression

noise-to-harmonics ratio (NHR) of 0.11, and voice turbulence index (VTI) of 0.031. Her maximum phonation time (MPT) was 20.1 s. Laryngeal endoscopic examination revealed bilateral Type 1 vocal fold Reinke's edema (RE).

The patient underwent an office-based steroid injection into both vocal folds using a 25-gauge flexible needle (Fig. 6.1a, b). The procedure was tolerated well by the patient with no complications noted.

On follow-up 4 weeks later, the patient had an improvement in her voice quality. Her VHI-10 score dropped to 2. Acoustic analysis revealed an increase in the F0 to 163.63 Hz and in HP to 155.5 Hz. Laryngeal examination showed almost complete disease regression (Fig. 6.1c).

6.2 Case 2

A 24-year-old man, a heavy smoker, presented to the clinic with loss of range, sore throat, and vocal fatigue. The patient had a positive history of voice abuse and denied any history of allergy or reflux disease. The patient also reported difficulty in breathing. His Voice Handicap Index-10 (VHI-10) score was 16. Acoustic analysis showed a fundamental frequency (F0) of 136.71 Hz, habitual pitch (HP) of

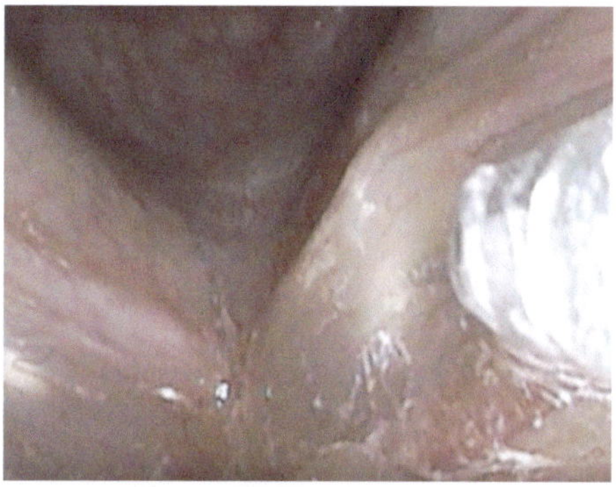

Fig. 6.2 An endoscopic view of the larynx showing a steroid injection into the RE of the right vocal fold

131.98 Hz, jitter of 0.53, shimmer of 1.67, noise-to-harmonics ratio (NHR) of 0.113, and voice turbulence index (VTI) of 0.025. His maximum phonation time (MPT) was 20.73 s. Laryngeal flexible endoscopic examination showed bilateral Reinke's edema (RE).

The patient underwent office-based steroid injection of methylprednisolone (0.3 ml) into the right vocal fold and 0.2 ml into the left vocal fold. The procedure was performed via the transnasal approach using the 25-gauge flexible needle (Fig. 6.2). The procedure was well tolerated by the patient with no complications noted.

On follow-up 6 weeks later, the patient had marked improvement in his voice quality. His VHI-10 score dropped to 7 and improvement in his acoustic parameters. Laryngeal examination revealed complete regression of the edema.

6.3 Case 3

A 56-year-old woman, a heavy smoker, presented to the voice clinic with hoarseness of a few months' duration. She denied any history of allergy or reflux disease. Her Voice Handicap Index-10 (VHI-10) score was 4. Auditory perceptual evaluation revealed grade 2 dysphonia. Acoustic analysis showed a fundamental frequency (F0) of 209 Hz and a habitual pitch (HP) of 148.39 Hz. Her maximum phonation time (MPT) was 9.86 s. Laryngeal flexible endoscopic evaluation showed a type 1 Reinke's edema (RE) of the right vocal fold and a small keratosis on the left vocal fold (Fig. 6.3a).

The patient underwent an office-based steroid injection. Using the transnasal approach, 0.2 cc of dexamethasone (8 mg/2 ml) was injected into Reinke's edema of the right vocal fold (Fig. 6.3b). The procedure was tolerated well by the patient with no complications noted.

On follow-up 4 weeks later, the patient had marked improvement in her voice quality. Her VHI-10 score dropped to 1. Acoustic analysis showed an increase in the F0 to 213.46 Hz, in HP to 171.41 Hz. There was also an increase in her MPT to 12.65 s. Laryngeal examination revealed partial disease regression.

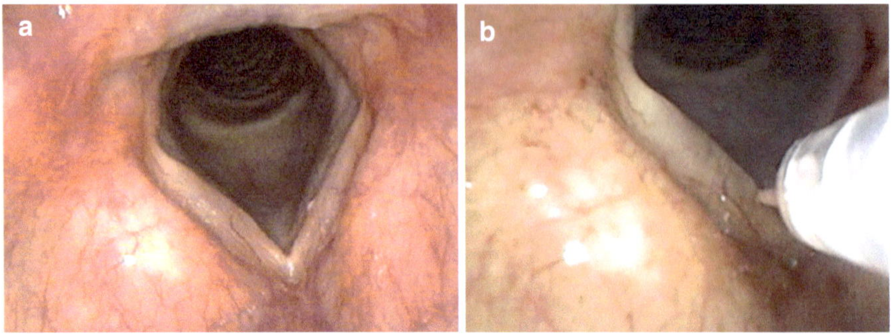

Fig. 6.3 (**a**) An endoscopic view of the larynx showing right vocal fold RE. Note a small keratotic lesion on the free edge of the left vocal fold. (**b**) An endoscopic view of the larynx showing the needle directed toward the right vocal fold RE

6.4 Case 4

A 47-year-old woman, smoker, presented to the voice clinic with hoarseness and shortness of breath following a thyroidectomy a few years ago. The patient denied any history of voice abuse, allergy or reflux disease. Her Voice Handicap Index-10 (VHI-10) score was 28. Acoustic analysis showed a fundamental frequency (F0) of 192 Hz, habitual pitch (HP) of 160.35 Hz, jitter of 1.15, shimmer of 3.07, noise-to-harmonics ratio (NHR) of 0.131, voice turbulence index (VTI) of 0.062. Her maximum phonation time (MPT) was 5.5 s. Laryngeal flexible endoscopy revealed bilateral vocal fold Reinke's edema (RE), left vocal fold paralysis, and right vocal fold paresis (Fig. 6.4a).

The patient underwent transnasal office-based steroid injection (0.1 cc of dexamethasone (8 mg/2 ml)) into the Reinke's edema of the right vocal fold using the 25-gauge flexible needle. The patient also underwent botulinum toxin injection 2.5 IU into each vocal fold. The procedure was tolerated well by the patient with no complications noted (Fig. 6.4b).

On follow-up 4 weeks later, the patient had a slight improvement in her voice quality. Her VHI-10 score dropped to 23. There was an increase in her MPT to 12 s. Laryngeal examination revealed a widening of the glottis and partial regression of the RE on the right side (Fig. 6.4c).

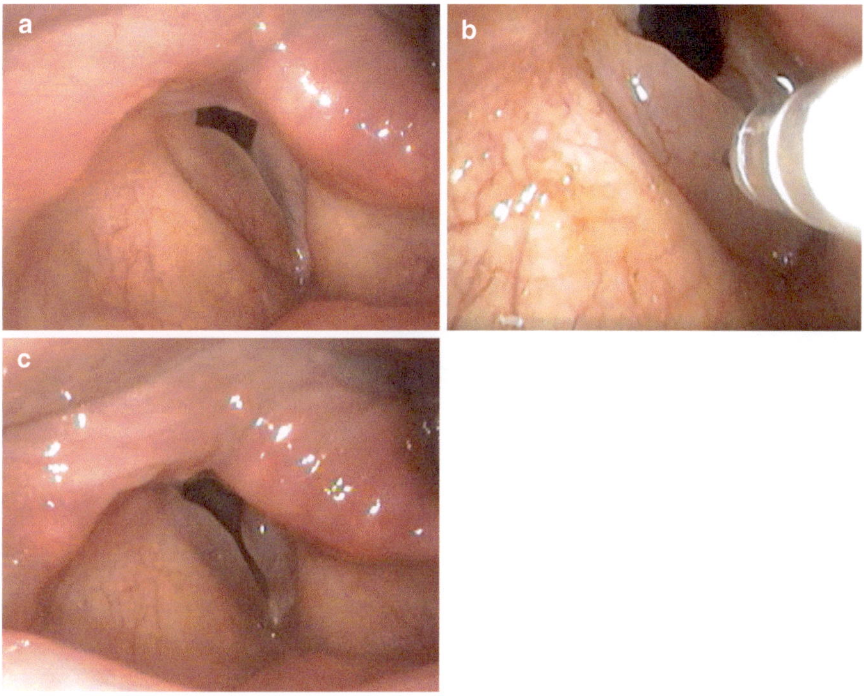

Fig. 6.4 (**a**) An endoscopic view of the larynx showing bilateral vocal fold RE with narrowing of the airway. (**b**) An endoscopic view of the larynx showing right vocal fold intralesional steroid injection. (**c**) An endoscopic view of the larynx 4 weeks after the injection showing partial disease regression

6.5 Case 5

A 30-year-old woman presented to the voice clinic with intermittent hoarseness that was worsening over time. The patient denied any history of smoking, phonotrauma, allergy or reflux disease. She was previously treated with oral steroids. Her Voice Handicap Index-10 (VHI-10) score was 21. Acoustic analysis showed a fundamental frequency (F0) of 180.4 Hz, habitual pitch (HP) of 216.53 Hz, jitter of 1.31, shimmer of 3.73, noise-to-harmonics ratio (NHR) of 0.127, and voice turbulence index (VTI) of 0.061. Her maximum phonation time (MPT) was 8.18 s. Laryngeal flexible endoscopic evaluation revealed bilateral vocal fold Reinke's edema (RE) (Fig. 6.5a, b).

The patient underwent an office-based steroid injection. The procedure was well tolerated by the patient with no complications noted (Fig. 6.5c).

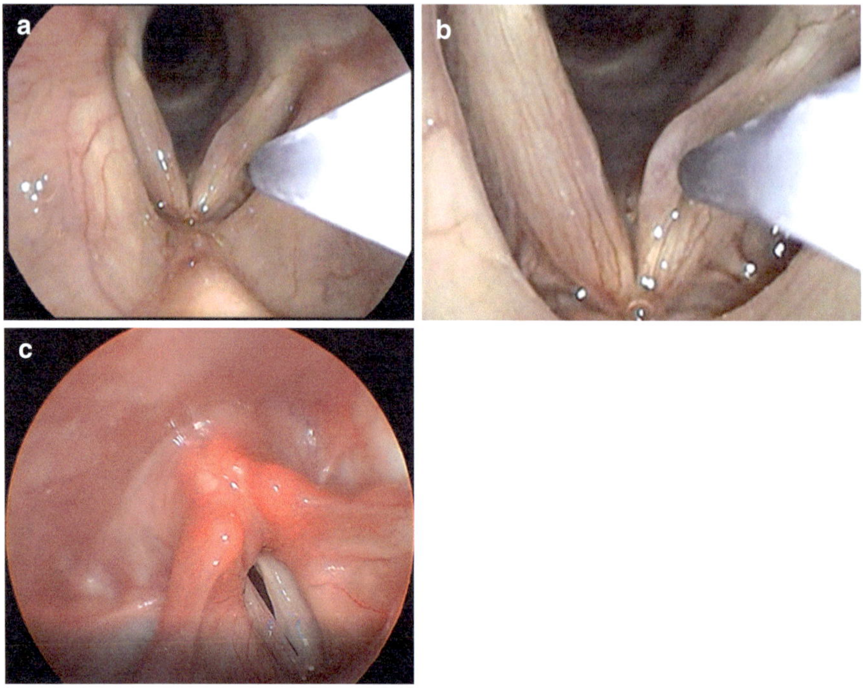

Fig. 6.5 (**a**) An endoscopic view of the larynx showing bilateral vocal fold RE type 1. (**b**) An endoscopic view of the larynx showing ILSI of the left vocal fold RE. (**c**) An endoscopic view of the larynx 3 months later showing localized edema of the left vocal fold and RE of the right vocal fold

On follow-up 3 months later, her VHI-10 score dropped to 8. Acoustic analysis revealed an increase in the F0 to 195.51 Hz. Laryngeal examination revealed partial disease regression. The patient was advised to undergo a second office-based steroids injection.

6.6 Case 6

A 49-year-old man, a heavy smoker, presented to the voice clinic with hoarseness of a few weeks' duration. The patient had a positive history of voice abuse and denied any history of allergy or reflux disease. His Voice Handicap Index-10 (VHI-10) score was 10. Acoustic analysis revealed a fundamental frequency (F0) of 78.94 Hz, a habitual pitch (HP) of 90 Hz, jitter of 1.17, shimmer of 6.87, noise-to-harmonics ratio (NHR) of 0.143, and voice turbulence index (VTI) of 0.05. His maximum phonation time (MPT) was 5.55 s. Laryngeal flexible endoscopic evaluation revealed bilateral type 1 Reinke's edema (RE) vocal fold.

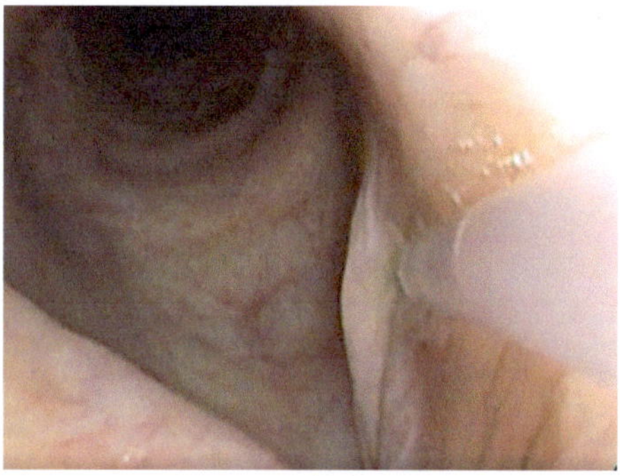

Fig. 6.6 An endoscopic view of the larynx showing ILSI of the left vocal fold RE

The patient underwent an office-based steroid injection. 0.3 ml of Dexamethasone (1 mg/1 ml) was injected into the Reinke's edema on each vocal fold using the 25-gauge flexible needle via the transnasal approach (Fig. 6.6). The procedure was well tolerated by the patient with no complications noted.

On follow-up 4 weeks later, the patient had marked improvement in his voice quality. His VHI-10 score dropped to 2. Acoustic analysis revealed a decrease in the F0 to 73.05 Hz, in shimmer to 5.3, and in the NHR to 0.135. There was an increase in the HP to 100 Hz. There was also an increase in the MPT to 9.35 s. Laryngeal examination revealed a marked reduction in Reinke's edema.

6.7 Case 7

A 69-year-old man, heavy smoker, presented to the voice clinic with hoarseness and mild dyspnea. The patient denied any history of allergy or reflux diseases. His Voice Handicap Index-10 (VHI-10) score was 10. Acoustic analysis showed a fundamental frequency (F0) of 127 Hz, habitual pitch (HP) of 112.1 Hz, jitter of 1.069, shimmer of 4.84, noise-to-harmonics ratio (NHR) of 0.142, and voice turbulence index (VTI) of 0.059. His maximum phonation time (MPT) was 5.82 s. Laryngeal examination showed bilateral vocal fold Reinke's Edema (RE).

The patient underwent office-based steroid injection. A total of 0.1 cc of Dexamethasone (8 mg/2 m) was injected into each vocal fold using a 25-gauge flexible needle. The injection was made via the transnasal approach (Fig. 6.7). The procedure was tolerated well by the patient with no complications noted.

On follow-up 4 weeks later, the patient had marked improvement in his breathing and voice quality. His VHI-10 score dropped to 1. Acoustic analysis showed an increase in the F0 to 137.36 Hz. Laryngeal examination revealed significant bilateral disease regression.

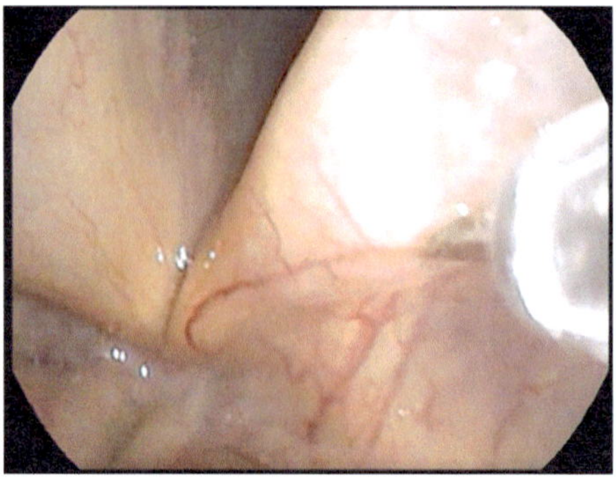

Fig. 6.7 An endoscopic view of the larynx showing the insertion of a 25-gauge needle into the left vocal fold's Reinke's edema. Note the edema and the increase in vascularity at the site of the injection

6.8 Case 8

A 57-year-old woman presented to the voice clinic with hoarseness of a few months' duration. The patient had a positive history of smoking and denied any history of allergy or reflux disease. Her Voice Handicap Index-10 (VHI-10) score was 32. Acoustic analysis revealed a fundamental frequency (F0) of 137.29 Hz, a habitual pitch (HP) of 222.59 Hz, jitter of 3, shimmer of 12.1, noise-to-harmonics ratio (NHR) of 0.452, and voice turbulence index (VTI) of 0.314. Her maximum phonation time (MPT) was 5.77 s. Her Dyspnea Severity Index (DSI) was 39. Laryngeal examination showed bilateral vocal fold Reinke's edema.

The patient underwent office-based intralesional steroid injection via the transnasal approach using a 25-gauge flexible needle. A total of 0.1 cc of dexamethasone (8 mg/2 ml) was injected into the left vocal fold, and 0.25 cc was injected into the right vocal fold. The procedure was tolerated well by the patient with no complications noted.

On follow-up 2 months later, the patient reported mild improvement in her voice quality. Endoscopic evaluation revealed partial regression of the lesion (Fig. 6.8a). The patient underwent a second office-based intralesional steroid injection using the 25-gauge flexible needle. A total of 0.3 cc of dexamethasone (8 mg/2 ml) was injected into each vocal fold (Fig. 6.8b).

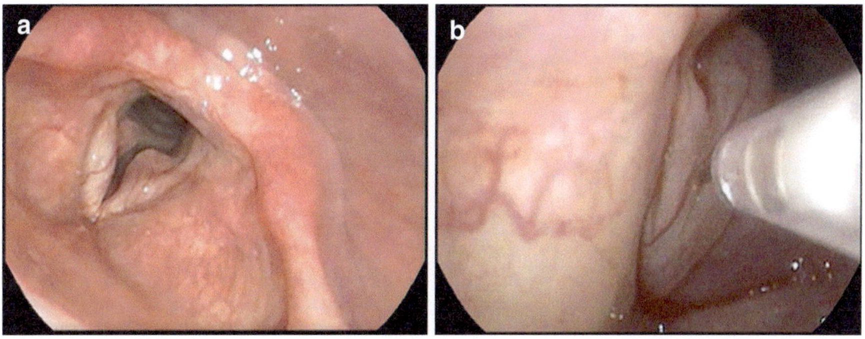

Fig. 6.8 (**a**) Laryngeal examination following the first intralesional steroid injection (ILSI) showing left vocal fold RE and right vocal fold polypoid mass. (**b**) An endoscopic view of the larynx showing steroid injection into the right vocal fold

On follow-up 6 weeks later, the patient reported marked improvement in her voice quality and breathing. Her VHI-10 score dropped to 16. Her DSI score dropped to 24. Acoustic analysis showed an increase in F0 to 250.64 Hz, and a decrease in the jitter to 1.571, in shimmer to 5.68, in NHR to 0.151, and in VTI to 0.089. Laryngeal examination showed significant regression in of the lesions.

6.9 Case 9

A 42-year-old woman presented to the voice clinic with hoarseness of a few months' duration. The patient had a positive history of voice abuse and reflux disease. Her Voice Handicap Index-10 (VHI-10) score was 7. Stroboscopic examination revealed localized vocal folds edema, more so on the left side (Fig. 6.9a).

The patient underwent office-based intralesional steroid injection using a 25-gauge flexible needle that was introduced into the working channel of a flexible nasopharyngoscope. A total of 0.2 cc of dexamethasone was injected into the left vocal fold, and 0.15 cc was injected into the right vocal fold (Fig. 6.9b). The procedure was tolerated well by the patient with no complications noted.

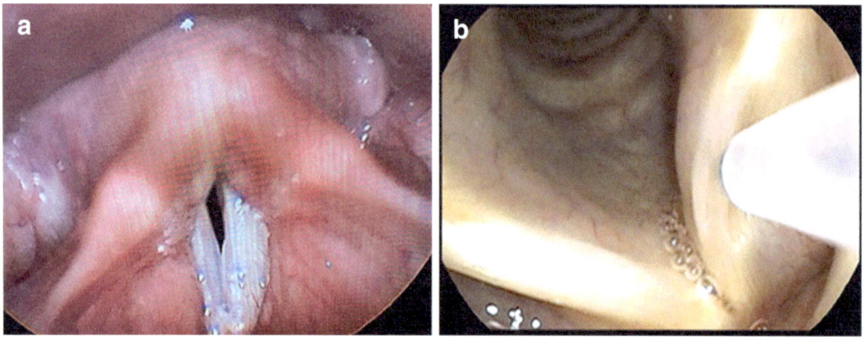

Fig. 6.9 (**a**) A stroboscopic view of the larynx showing localized vocal fold edema, more so on the left vocal fold. Note the incomplete closure of the vocal folds during phonation. (**b**) An endoscopic view of the larynx showing left vocal fold steroid injection

6.10 Case 10

A 34-year-old man presented to the voice clinic with hoarseness of a few months' duration. The patient had a positive history of smoking, voice abuse, and reflux disease. He denied any history of allergy. His Voice Handicap Index-10 (VHI-10) score was 7. Acoustic analysis revealed a habitual pitch (HP) of 169.16 Hz, jitter 0.44, shimmer 2.53, noise-to-harmonics ratio (NHR) of 0.135, voice turbulence index (VTI) of 0.095. His maximum phonation time (MPT) was 13.3 s. Laryngeal examination showed bilateral vocal fold Reinke's Edema (Fig. 6.10a).

The patient underwent office-based intralesional steroid injection using a 25-gauge flexible needle via the transnasal approach. A total of 0.1 cc of dexamethasone (8 mg/2 ml) was injected into each vocal fold (Fig. 6.10b). The procedure was tolerated well by the patient with no complications noted.

On follow-up 4 months later, the patient reported marked improvement in his voice quality. His VHI-10 score was 11. Acoustic analysis showed a decrease in the perturbation parameters (jitter dropped to 0.15 and shimmer dropped to 1.76). Laryngeal examination revealed significant regression of the RE with minimal residual disease seen on the left vocal fold. The patient was advised to undergo a second office-based steroid injection.

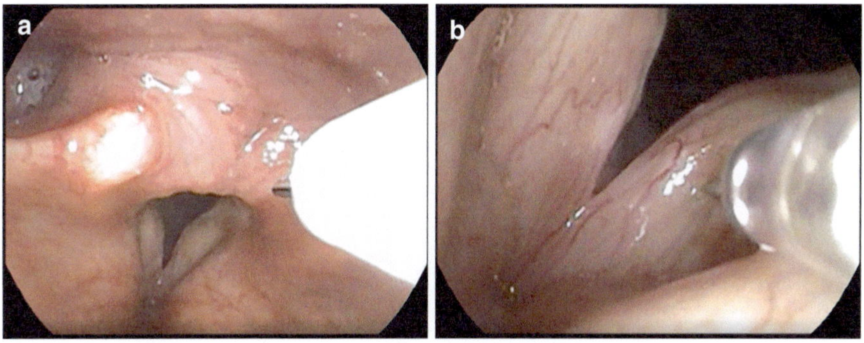

Fig. 6.10 (**a**) An endoscopic view of the larynx showing bilateral Reinke's edema. (**b**) Intra-operative view of the larynx showing intralesional steroid injection on the left side

6.11 Case 11

A 76-year-old woman presented to the voice clinic with hoarseness of a few weeks' duration. The patient had a positive history of voice abuse and reflux disease. She was a former smoker. Her Voice Handicap Index-10 (VHI-10) score was 24. Acoustic analysis showed a fundamental frequency (F0) of 118.51 Hz, habitual pitch (HP) of 116.09 Hz, jitter of 0.873, shimmer of 2.56, noise-to-harmonics ratio (NHR) of 0.134, and voice turbulence index (VTI) of 0.036. Her maximum phonation time (MPT) was 7.81 s. Laryngeal examination revealed bilateral Reinke's edema type 1, and a yellowish discoloration of the left vocal fold suggestive of recent bleeding (Fig. 6.11a).

The patient underwent office-based intralesional steroid injection using a 25-gauge flexible needle that was introduced into the working channel of a flexible nasopharyngoscope (Fig. 6.11b). A total of 0.1 cc of dexamethasone (8 mg/2 ml) was injected into each vocal fold. The procedure was tolerated well by the patient with no complications noted.

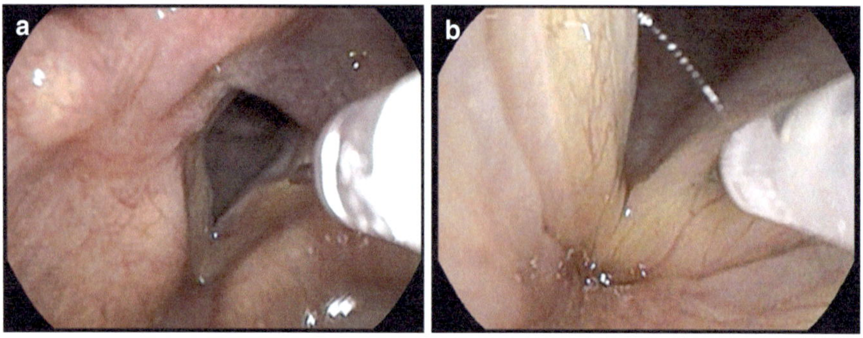

Fig. 6.11 (**a**) An endoscopic view of the larynx showing bilateral RE with a yellowish discoloration of the left vocal fold suggestive of a recent submucosal hemorrhage. (**b**) An endoscopic view of the larynx showing a left vocal fold steroid injection

6.12 Case 12

A 35-year-old singer presented to the voice clinic with hoarseness of a few months' duration. He reported loss of high notes, difficulty transitioning between registers, and inability to sustain a note. The patient had a positive history of smoking, voice abuse, and reflux disease. He denied any history of allergy. His Voice Handicap Index-10 (VHI-10) score was 4. Acoustic analysis revealed a fundamental frequency (F0) of 102.1 Hz, habitual pitch (HP) of 96.73 Hz, jitter of 0.42, shimmer of 2.3, noise-to-harmonics ratio (NHR) of 0.14, and voice turbulence index (VTI) of 0.038. His maximum phonation time (MPT) was 24.07 s. Laryngeal examination showed localized edema of the right vocal fold (Fig. 6.12a). Patient was advised voice rest and vocal hygiene therapy, followed by vocal fold steroid injection in case of no improvement.

The patient underwent office-based intralesional steroid injection using A 25-gauge flexible needle (Fig. 6.12b). The procedure was tolerated well by the patient with no complications noted. On follow-up 3 weeks later, the patient reported marked improvement in his voice quality. His VHI-10 score was 0.

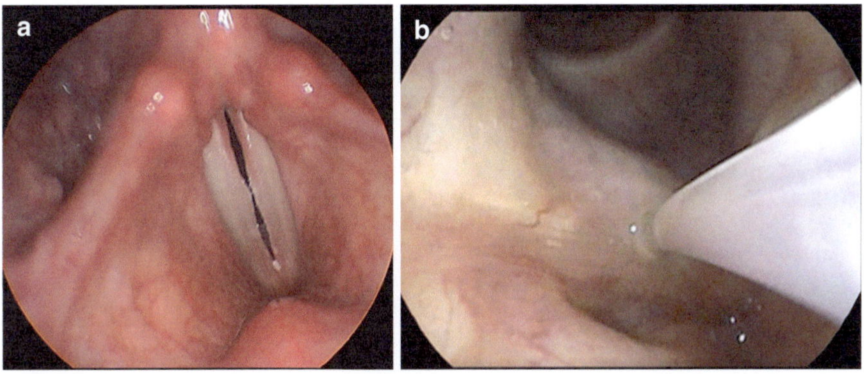

Fig. 6.12 (**a**) An endoscopic view of the larynx showing localized edema of the right vocal fold. (**b**) An intra-operative view of right vocal fold intralesional steroid injection

References

1. Druck Sant'Anna G, Mauri M. Use of the microdebrider for Reinke's edema surgery. Laryngoscope. 2000;110(12):2114–6.
2. Marcotullio D, Magliulo G, Pezone T. Reinke's edema and risk factors: clinical and histopathologic aspects. Am J Otolaryngol. 2002;23(2):81–4.
3. Lechien JR, Saussez S, Nacci A, et al. Association between laryngopharyngeal reflux and benign vocal folds lesions: a systematic review. Laryngoscope. 2019;129(9):E329–41.
4. Courey MS, Shohet JA, Scott MA, Ossoff RH. Immunohistochemical characterization of benign laryngeal lesions. Ann Otol Rhinol Laryngol. 1996;105(7):525–31.
5. Silva F, Legou T, Champsaur P, Giovanni A, Lagier A. Contact pressure between the vocal folds in Reinke's edema: experimental observations on an excised human larynx. J Voice. 2021;35(6):931.e15–20.
6. Kravos A, Hočevar-Boltežar I, Geršak K. Serum levels of sex hormones in males with Reinke's edema. Eur Arch Otorrinolaringol. 2013;270(1):233–8.
7. Pastuszek P, Krecicki T, Zalesska-Krecicka M, Jeleń M, Rak J, Krajewska B. Histological and electron microscopic investigation of Reinke's edema. Pol J Pathol. 2003;54(1):61–4.
8. Sakae FA, Imamura R, Sennes LU, et al. Disarrangement of collagen fibers in Reinke's edema. Laryngoscope. 2008;118(8):1500–3.
9. Sakae FA, Imamura R, Sennes LU, et al. Elastic fibers in Reinke's edema. Ann Otol Rhinol Laryngol. 2010;119(9):609–14.
10. Gray SD, Hammond E, Hanson DF. Benign pathologic responses of the larynx. Ann Otol Rhinol Laryngol. 1995;104(1):13–8.
11. Hirschi SD, Gray SD, Thibeault SL. Fibronectin: an interesting vocal fold protein. J Voice. 2002;16(3):310–6.
12. Hamdan AL, Khalifee E, Abi Akl PR, Ghanem A, El Hage A. Pathogenic role of Reinke's edema in snoring and obstructive sleep apnea. J Voice. 2020;34(3):456–9.
13. Tan M, Bryson PC, Pitts C, et al. Clinical grading of Reinke's edema. Laryngoscope. 2017;127(10):2310–3.
14. Watanabe T, Kaneko K, Sakaguchi K, Takahashi H. Vocal-fold vibration of patients with Reinke's edema observed using high-speed digital imaging. Auris Nasus Larynx. 2016;43(6):654–7.

15. Zalesska-Krecicka M, Krecicki T, Cyganek P. A clinical study of Reinke's edema. Otolaryngol Pol. 1993;47(2):153–7.
16. Courey MS, Stone RE, Gardner GM, et al. Endoscopic vocal fold microflap: a three-year experience. Ann Otol Rhinol Laryngol. 1995;104:267–73.
17. Sataloff RT, Spiegel JR, Heuer RJ, et al. Laryngeal mini-microflap: a new technique and reassessment of the microflap saga. J Voice. 1995;9:198–204.
18. Schyberg YM, Bork KH, Sørensen MK, Rasmussen N. "Cold-steel" phonosurgery of Reinke edema evaluated by the multidimensional voice program. J Voice. 2018;32(2):244–8.
19. Nielsen VM, Højslet PE, Karlsmose M. Surgical treatment of Reinke's oedema (long-term results). J Laryngol Otol. 1986;100(2):187–90.
20. Hamdan AL, Abi Zeid Daou C, Ghanem A, A R Feghali P, Hosri J, Sataloff RT. Office-based laser therapy in Reinke's edema: a systematic review and meta-analysis. J Voice. 2025;39(3):799–805.
21. Tateya I, Omori K, Kojima H, Hirano S, Kaneko K, Ito J. Steroid injection for Reinke's edema using fiberoptic laryngeal surgery. Acta Otolaryngol. 2003;123(3):417–20.
22. Takahashi S, Kanazawa T, Hasegawa T, Hirosaki M, Komazawa D, Konomi U, Nimura Y, Sakaguchi Y, Nozawa M, Yamauchi T, Watanabe Y. Comparison of therapeutic effects of steroid injection by benign vocal fold lesion type. Acta Otolaryngol. 2021;141(11):1005–13.
23. Hamdan AL, Hosri J, Daou CAZ, Ghzayel L, Hadi J, Saab MB, Kasti M, Mourad M. Office-based steroid injection for benign lesions of the vocal folds: case series and review of the literature. J Voice. 2024:S0892-1997(24)00095-X.

7 Office-Based Steroid Injection for Vocal Fold Cysts

Vocal fold mucus retention cysts are benign lesions of the vocal folds that arise from obstruction of the excretory duct of mucus glands. They are a rare cause of hoarseness in adults and children. Affected patients present with a change in voice quality, alteration in pitch, and voice fatigue. Singers may complain of volume disturbance, difficulty transitioning between registers, contracted vocal range, and loss of the high notes [1, 2]. On laryngeal examination, vocal fold mucus retention cysts appear as submucosal yellowish lesions that vary in size. A reactive lesion on the contralateral vocal fold may be seen. Stroboscopy shows asymmetry in vocal fold vibration, with a decrease or absence of mucosal waves at the site of the lesion. Incomplete closure of the vocal folds during phonation may be observed if the lesion is at the free edge of the vocal fold [3, 4].

The treatment of vocal fold mucus retention cysts is surgical. Early intervention is often recommended to avoid scar formation [5]. Microlaryngeal surgery is routinely performed in the operating room and consists of "en bloc" removal of the lesion to prevent recurrence. Diligent dissection of the wall of the cyst and sparing of the overlying mucosa are advocated [6–8]. Marsupialization of the cyst has also been reported as an alternative treatment option to "en bloc" resection. The term "wide-opening method" has been described by Chang et al. to denote a surgical technique whereby the medial wall of the cyst and the overlying mucosa are removed. The authors recommended the "wide-opening method" for large cysts, the enucleation of which—using the standard surgical technique—might be very challenging [9].

With the advances in technology and the shift of laryngeal surgery from the operating room to the clinic, office-based therapy for vocal fold benign lesions—including cysts—has gained popularity among otolaryngologists, particularly for patients at high risk for general anesthesia. A commonly performed office-based treatment

---

Supplementary Information The online version contains supplementary material available at https://doi.org/10.1007/978-3-032-05235-3_7.

A. L. Hamdan, *Atlas of Office-based Laryngeal Steroid Injection*,
https://doi.org/10.1007/978-3-032-05235-3_7

option is laser therapy. Using the laser in a contact mode, the cyst wall is incised to allow extrusion of the cyst content. The laser glass fiber may be used to clean the surgical bed. Hamdan et al. reported the successful use of a thulium laser in three cases of vocal fold cysts under local anesthesia. All patients had complete disease regression with no recurrence noted on follow-up a year later. The same authors reported two other cases of vocal fold mucus retention cysts—and one cases of vocal fold pseudocyst—treated in-office using the blue laser. There was an improvement in both subjective and objective voice outcome measures following treatment [10]. Gao et al. described the use of a potassium titanyl laser for marsupialization of four cases of vocal fold mucus retention cysts. All patients improved after surgery, and no recurrence was noted [11].

Another effective office-based treatment modality for vocal fold cysts is steroid injection. Wu et al. reported their experience with office-based steroid injections for vocal fold mucus retention cysts in 57 patients and noted significant disease regression in 84% of the cases. The authors used a 1:1 mixture of dexamethasone and triamcinolone injected intralesionally via the transoral or transnasal approach. The disease regression on laryngeal endoscopy 2 months later was associated with a significant drop in the VHI-10 score by ten points, a significant improvement in the auditory perceptual rating, and a significant decrease in perturbation parameters. The decrease in the size of the lesion also led to a significant increase in the maximum phonation time by almost 2.1 s. Nevertheless, one-third of their study group had recurrence on follow-up 2 months or more later. The short-term recurrence was ascribed to the re-accumulation of mucus within the cyst following the injection [12]. Similarly, Wang et al. reported significant disease regression in 30 cases of vocal fold mucus retention cysts treated in-office with intralesional steroid injections. Complete and/or partial improvement on examination was noted in 29% and 76% of the cases, respectively. The disease regression was associated with significant improvement in objective voice measures [13]. Mortensen and Woo reported their experience with in-office steroid injections in 34 patients with various vocal fold pathologies and noted significant improvement in 82% of the cases. The improvement was observed mostly in the cases of vocal fold polyps and nodules—and less in vocal fold scars. The two patients, one with a vocal fold pseudocyst and the other with a polyp-cyst, had no improvement and needed further treatment [14].

7.1 Case 1

A 39-year-old woman presented to the voice clinic with a history of hoarseness of a few months' duration. She had a positive history of smoking, reflux disease, and voice overuse. She denied any history of allergy. Her Voice Handicap Index-10 (VHI-10) score on the presentation was 16. Acoustic analysis revealed a fundamental frequency (F0) of 147.94 Hz, habitual pitch (HP) of 154.77 Hz, jitter of 0.053, shimmer of 1.84, noise-to-harmonics ratio (NHR) of 0.118, and a Voice Turbulence Index (VTI) of 0.046. Aerodynamic analysis showed a maximum phonation time

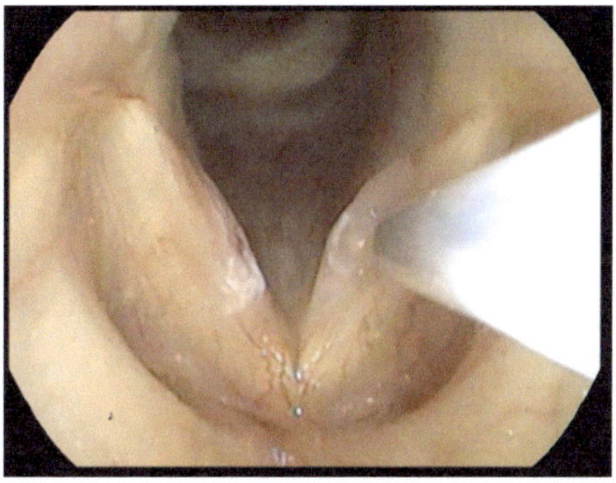

Fig. 7.1 An endoscopic view of the larynx showing edema of the left vocal fold with a well-delineated cyst at the free edge and a reactive lesion on the contralateral vocal fold. Note the insertion of the needle at the site of the lesion

(MPT) of 9.29 s. Laryngeal endoscopic examination revealed edema of the left vocal fold with a well-delineated cyst at the free edge and a reactive lesion on the contralateral vocal fold.

The patient underwent an office-based steroid injection under local anesthesia (Fig. 7.1). The procedure was tolerated well by the patient, with no complications noted.

The patient presented for a follow-up a year and a half later. She reported marked improvement in her voice quality. Laryngeal endoscopic examination revealed complete regression of the lesions.

7.2 Case 2

A 63-year-old woman presented to the voice clinic with hoarseness of a few months' duration. The patient had a positive history of smoking and voice abuse and denied any history of reflux disease or allergy. Her Voice Hand cap Index-10 (VHI-10) score was 16. Acoustic analysis revealed a fundamental frequency (F0) of 267.25 Hz, habitual pitch (HP) of 250.3 Hz, jitter: 1.14, shimmer 3.48, noise-to-harmonics ratio (NHR) of 0.147, and voice turbulence index (VTI) of 0.036. Her maximum phonation time (MPT) was 12.46 s. Flexible laryngoscopy showed a left vocal fold cyst with a reactive lesion on the opposite side (Fig. 7.2a).

The patient underwent an office-based intralesional steroid injection under local anesthesia. A 25-gauge needle was inserted into the working channel of the nasopharyngoscope, and 0.2 cc of dexamethasone (8 mg/2 ml) was injected into the left vocal fold cyst. The procedure was tolerated well by the patient with no complications noted (Fig. 7.2b–d; Video 7.1).

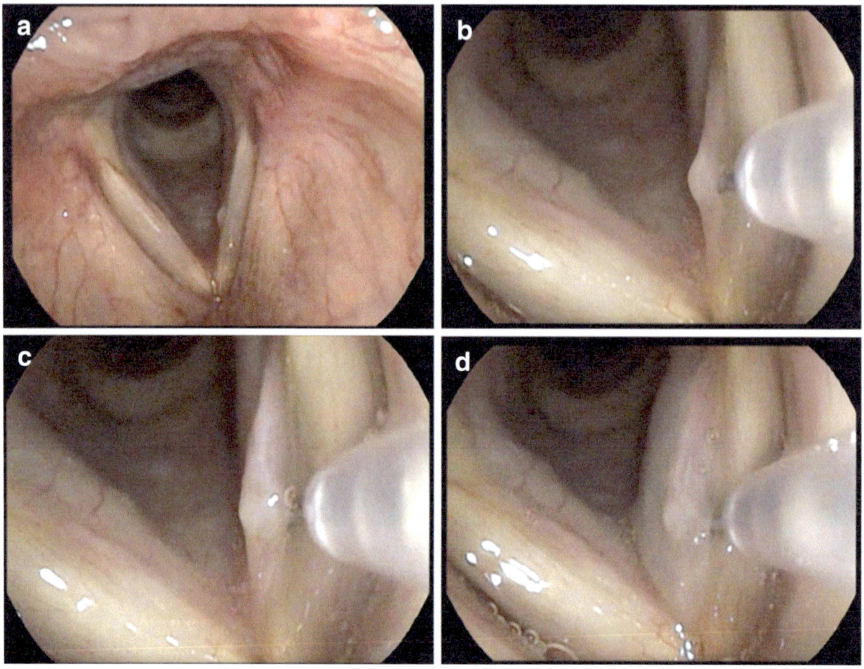

Fig. 7.2 (**a**) An endoscopic view of the larynx showing a left vocal fold cyst. (**b**) Intraoperative view showing the insertion of the needle within the cyst. (**c**) An endoscopic view of the larynx showing steroid solution filling the Reinke's space. (**d**) An endoscopic view of the larynx toward the end of the procedure

References

1. Martins RH, Santana MF, Tavares EL. Vocal cysts: clinical, endoscopic, and surgical aspects. J Voice. 2011;25(1):107–10.
2. Swain SK. Vocal fold cyst: a narrative review. J Clin Sci Res. 2024;13(1):52–8.
3. Rosen CA, Gartner-Schmidt J, Hathaway B, et al. A nomenclature paradigm for benign mid-membranous vocal fold lesions. Laryngoscope. 2012;122(6):1335–41.
4. Sataloff RT. Structural abnormalities of the larynx. In: Sataloff RT, editor. Professional voice: the science and art of clinical care. 4th ed. San Diego: Plural; 2017. p. 1533–86.
5. Woo P. Office-based laryngeal procedures. Otolaryngol Clin N Am. 2006;39(1):111–33.
6. Sataloff RT, Spiegel JR, Heuer RJ, Baroody MM, Emerich KA, Hawkshaw MJ, Rosen DC. Laryngeal mini-microflap: a new technique and reassessment of the microflap saga. J Voice. 1995;9(2):198–204.
7. Altman KW. Vocal fold masses. Otolaryngol Clin N Am. 2007;40(5):1091–108.
8. Reder LS, Franco RA. Benign vocal fold lesions. Pract Laryngol. 2015;27.
9. Chang HP, Chang SY. An alternative surgical procedure for the treatment of vocal fold retention cyst. Otolaryngol Head Neck Surg. 2003;128(4):470–7.

10. Hamdan AL, Abou Raji Feghali P, Hosri J, Ghanem A, Alam E. Office-based laser therapy for vocal fold cyst: a promising alternative therapy using the 445 nm blue laser. J Voice. 2023;S0892-1997(23)00172-8.
11. Gao WZ, Abu-Ghanem S, Reder LS, Amin M, Johns MM. A novel approach to vocal fold mucous retention cysts: awake KTP laser-assisted marsupialization. J Voice. 2022;36(4):570–3.
12. Wu PH, Cheng PW, Lin FC, Wang CT. Intralesional steroid injection as an alternative treatment for 57 patients of vocal fold mucus retention cysts. Clin Otolaryngol. 2018;43(5):1375–8.
13. Wang CT, Lai MS, Hsiao TY. Comprehensive outcome researches of intralesional steroid injection on benign vocal fold lesions. J Voice. 2015;29(5):578–87.
14. Mortensen M, Woo P. Office steroid injections of the larynx. Laryngoscope. 2006;116(10):1735–9.

8 Office-Based Steroid Injection for Vocal Process Granuloma

Vocal process granuloma is a benign lesion of the glottis commonly encountered in otolaryngology practice. It was first described by Chevalier Jackson in 1928 as a contact ulcer on the mucosal surface of the posterior larynx [1]. Since then, various other—terms such as contact granuloma, arytenoid granuloma, and pyogenic granuloma—have been described to denote the same laryngeal pathology.

The etiology of vocal process granuloma is complex. Several predisposing factors have been identified, the most common of which is reflux disease [2]. Animal studies have shown that vocal process granuloma can be induced by applying the gastroduodenal contents to the larynx [3]. To that end, the term "peptic granuloma" has been coined by many authors as an alternative to "contact granuloma" [4]. The retrograde movement of the acidic and nonacidic refluxate material into the posterior glottis instigates a cascade of inflammatory changes, leading to erythema, ulceration, and mass formation [5]. The etiologic role of reflux disease has been further substantiated by the patient's response to anti-reflux therapy in almost 50% of the cases [6].

Other causes of vocal process granuloma include infectious diseases of the upper airway, which can be bacterial, viral, or fungal. These result in mucositis, excess mucus production, and post-nasal drip—which can elicit cough and throat clearing. Phonotrauma, in the form of repetitive throat clearing or other forms of voice abuse, is also a risk factor for vocal process granuloma formation. The harsh striking of one vocal process against the other—a mechanism referred to as "Hammer and anvil,"—may incite or precipitate the development of these lesions [1].

Another form of trauma is laryngeal manipulation, such as following a difficult intubation. While introducing the endotracheal tube into the airway, injury to the mucosal lining of the posterior glottis, perichondrium, or arytenoid cartilages may

---

Supplementary Information The online version contains supplementary material available at https://doi.org/10.1007/978-3-032-05235-3_8.

A. L. Hamdan, *Atlas of Office-based Laryngeal Steroid Injection*, https://doi.org/10.1007/978-3-032-05235-3_8

occur. In 1994, Santos et al. reported several signs of post-intubation laryngeal injury, the most common of which were erythema and ulceration—present in 94% and 76% of the cases, respectively. Laryngeal granuloma was found in 44% of the cases [7]. It is important to note that vocal process granuloma may be associated with thickening of the underlying cartilage. Osteosclerosis may be seen on radiologic images—alluding to the significant depth of injury [8].

Other forms of granulomas of the posterior larynx are also seen following laser glottal widening procedures—such as posterior cordectomy or partial arytenoidectomy—for the treatment of bilateral vocal fold paralysis [9, 10].

Patients with vocal process granuloma may be asymptomatic or present with throat clearing, cough, globus pharyngeus, foreign body sensation, and change in voice quality. Less commonly reported symptoms are hemoptysis—in the case of an ulcerative lesion—and dyspnea, or shortness of breath—in the case of a large obstructive lesion. Flexible laryngoscopy reveals a mass in the posterior larynx, usually located on the medial and superior surface of the vocal process. The lesion can be ulcerative, fungating, polypoidal, or proliferative. The presence of such a lesion in the larynx is usually indicative of a vocal process granuloma. However, in cases of a high index of suspicion, other disease entities—such as granulomatous infectious lesions, inflammatory pseudo-tumors, hemangioma, angiofibroma, and squamous cell carcinoma—must be excluded. The need for a laryngeal biopsy should be considered in the context of the clinical presentation of the patient, and the presence of other risk factors—such as smoking or a positive family history of laryngeal cancer [11].

The treatment of vocal process granuloma is not singular. Management should be tailored based on the patient's history and clinical presentation. Various treatment options have been described in the literature, the most common being anti-reflux therapy. The management of reflux aims to prevent the retrograde movement of gastroduodenal contents into the laryngopharyngeal complex. Dietary behavioral modification—such as avoiding the intake of acidic food—is the first line of therapy. Lack of response to dietary behavioral modification should prompt the physician to initiate medical treatment—such as the intake of proton pump inhibitors and antacids. The use of adjunctive drug therapy, like antibiotics and steroids, has been described by some authors—with no clear consensus on its added value [12, 13]. Voice therapy has also been advocated in patients with hyperfunctional laryngeal behavior. Voice rest, elimination of bad phonatory habits, and relaxation exercises act in concert to reduce the harshness of the glottal attack and to decrease the collision intensity between the vocal folds during phonation.

Surgical excision of vocal process granuloma is usually reserved for patients who are refractory to treatment and/or in cases of a large lesion obstructing the airway. Other indications for surgery include the need to establish a histopathologic diagnosis in patients with suspicious lesions. Different surgical techniques have been described—ranging from superficial excision or ablation to removal of the entire lesion [12, 14]. Despite advances in instrumentation and the use of various surgical tools, the recurrence rate after surgical intervention remains high. Some predictors of recurrence include the type of vocalization, smoking, and alcohol consumption [15].

With the reform in laryngology practice towards office-based surgery, office-based procedures—such as intralesional steroid injection—have gained popularity among otolaryngologists. Intralesional steroid injection aims at delivering a high dosage of steroid within the vocal process granuloma while averting the adverse effects of systemic therapy. Intralesional steroid injection can be performed as a primary treatment modality or in combination with laryngeal botulinum toxin injection into one or more of the adductor muscles. The purpose of the injection is to induce temporary denervation of the adductor muscles, which allows healing of the injured mucosa.

Transthyroid botulinum toxin injection was first described by Nasri et al. [16] and has been adopted by many authors [16–21]. Various injection techniques have been described, and different adductor muscles can be injected. The most commonly used approaches are the thyrohyoid and cricothyroid approaches—with or without laryngeal electromyographic guidance [22, 23]. Another used approach is the transnasal approach. Using a flexible nasopharyngoscope with a working channel, a flexible 25-gauge needle is introduced and advanced toward the injection site [24]. Laryngeal botulinum toxin injection may also be performed via the peroral approach—using a curved needle that is introduced under visual guidance [25].

8.1 Case 1

A 39-year-old male patient presented to the voice clinic with neck pain and odynophonia. He denied any history of smoking, allergy, or reflux disease. His VHI-10 score at presentation was 9. Acoustic analysis revealed a fundamental frequency of 103.84 Hz, a habitual pitch of 104.12 Hz, a jitter of 0.37, a shimmer of 1.63, a noise-to-harmonics ratio of 0.14, and a voice turbulence index of 0.025. His maximum phonation time was 16.16 s. Laryngeal endoscopic examination showed a right vocal process granuloma (Fig. 8.1a).

The patient underwent office-based intralesional steroid injection via the thyrohyoid approach. A total of 0.3 cc of dexamethasone (8 mg/2 ml) was injected into the right vocal process granuloma (Fig. 8.1b). As an adjuvant therapy, 0.2 cc of botulinum toxin (5 IU) was injected into the interarytenoid muscle. The procedure was tolerated well by the patient, with no complications noted.

On follow-up 3 months later, the patient had complete disease regression. His VHI-10 dropped to 2. Acoustic analysis revealed a decrease in the noise-to-harmonics ratio to 0.07 and an increase in maximum phonation time to 18.9 s (Fig. 8.1c).

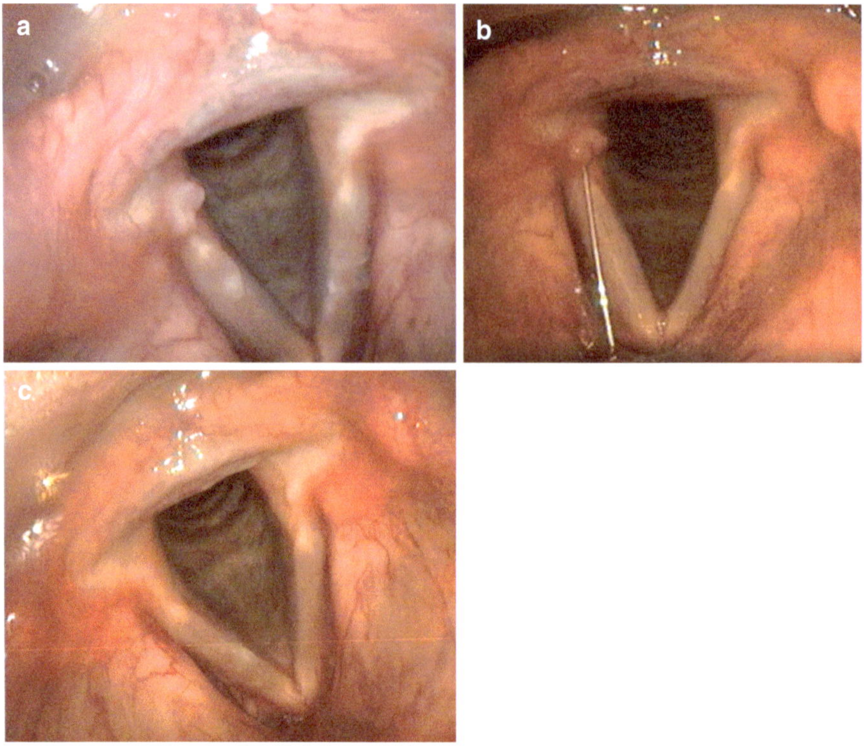

Fig. 8.1 (**a**) An endoscopic view showing a right vocal process granuloma. (**b**) An endoscopic view showing the tip of a 25-gauge needle inserted into the right vocal process granuloma. (**c**) An endoscopic view of the larynx 3 months after the procedure, revealing the complete regression of the process granuloma

8.2 Case 2

A 52-year-old man presented to the voice clinic with repetitive throat clearing and a globus sensation. The patient denied any history of smoking, phonotrauma, allergy, or reflux disease. His Voice Handicap Index-10 (VHI-10) score was 4. Acoustic analysis showed a fundamental frequency (F0) of 96.06 Hz, a habitual pitch (HP) of 93.88 Hz, a jitter of 0.2, a shimmer of 2.77, a noise-to-harmonics ratio (NHR) of 0.115, and a Voice Turbulence Index (VTI) of 0.029. His maximum phonation time (MPT) was 25.05 s. Laryngeal endoscopic examination revealed a right vocal cord process granuloma (Fig. 8.2a).

The patient underwent an office-based steroid injection into the right vocal process granuloma. A total of 0.2 cc of dexamethasone (8 mg/2 ml) was injected using a 25-gauge flexible needle—that was introduced through the thyrohyoid membrane (Fig. 8.2b). The procedure was tolerated well by the patient, with no complications noted.

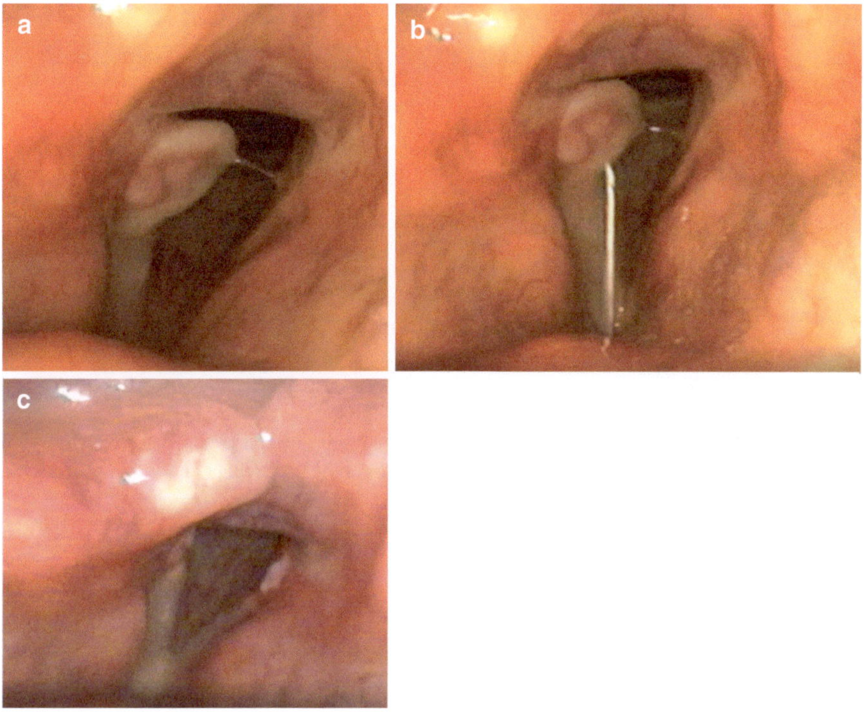

Fig. 8.2 (**a**) An endoscopic view of the larynx showing a right vocal process granuloma. (**b**) An endoscopic view showing the tip of a 25-gauge needle inserted into the right vocal process granuloma. (**c**) An endoscopic view of the larynx 2 months after the injection, showing almost complete regression of the right vocal process granuloma. Also note an ulceration on the medial surface of the left vocal process

On follow-up 8 weeks later, the patient had improvement in his symptoms. His VHI-10 score dropped to 2. Acoustic analysis showed an increase in the F0 to 99 Hz with no significant change in the other acoustic parameters. Laryngeal examination revealed almost complete regression of the lesion (Fig. 8.2c). The patient was advised to undergo voice therapy.

8.3 Case 3

A 24-year-old male patient presented to the clinic with a history of intermittent dyspnea. He had a positive history of reflux disease refractory to medical therapy using a proton pump inhibitor (PPI). The patient had no history of smoking or allergy. Flexible fiberoptic laryngoscopy revealed a right vocal process granuloma (Fig. 8.3a).

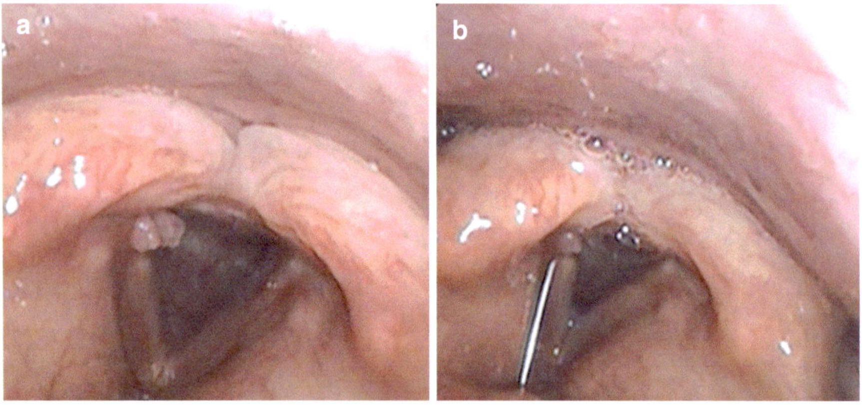

Fig. 8.3 (**a**) An endoscopic view of the larynx showing a right vocal process granuloma. (**b**) An intraoperative view of the larynx showing intralesional steroid injection. Note the tip of the needle at the base of the right vocal process granuloma

The patient underwent office-based intralesional steroid injection (ILSI) combined with botulinum toxin injection into the interarytenoid muscle—under local anesthesia (Fig. 8.3b, Video 8.1). The patient tolerated the procedure well with no complications.

8.4 Case 4

A 41-year-old man presented to the voice clinic with hoarseness and throat clearing of a few months' duration. He had a positive history of reflux disease. He denied any history of smoking, allergy, and phonotrauma. His voice handicap index (VHI-10) score on the presentation was 7. Acoustic analysis showed a Fundamental Frequency (F0) of 91.02 Hz, a Habitual Pitch of 99.07 Hz, a Jitter of 0.86, a Shimmer of 2.09, a noise-to-harmonics ratio (NHR) of 0.119, and a voice turbulence index (VTI) of 0.037. His maximum phonation time (MPT) was 16.02 s. Laryngeal endoscopic examination revealed a left vocal process granuloma (Fig. 8.4a).

The patient underwent office-steroid injection—under local anesthesia. Using a retrobulbar needle, 0.4 cc of dexamethasone (8 mg/2 ml) was injected into the left vocal process granuloma via the percutaneous approach. The procedure was well tolerated by the patient, with no complications noted (Fig. 8.4b).

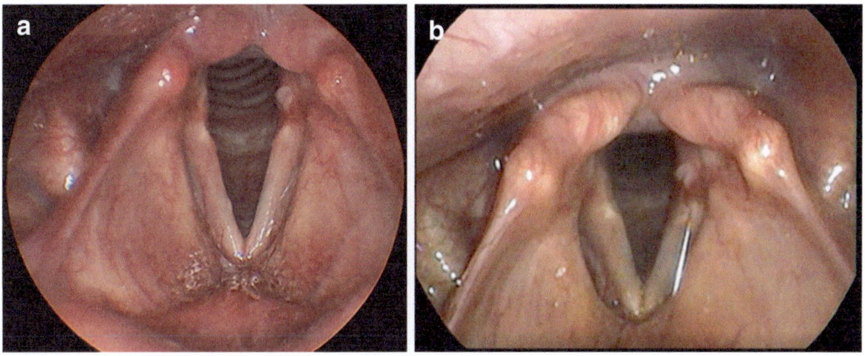

Fig. 8.4 (**a**) An endoscopic view of the larynx showing a left vocal process granuloma. (**b**) An intraoperative view of the larynx showing intralesional steroid injection. Note the tip of the needle at the base of the left vocal process granuloma

References

1. Jackson C, Jackson CL. Contact ulcer of the larynx. Arch Otolaryngol. 1935;22:1–15.
2. McFerran DJ, Abdullah V, Gallimore AP, Pringle MB, Croft CB. Vocal process granulomata. J Laryngol Otol. 1994;108:216–20.
3. Delahunty JE, Cherry J. Experimentally produced vocal cord granulomas. Laryngoscope. 1968;78:1941–7.
4. Miko TL. Peptic (contact ulcer) granuloma of the larynx. J Clin Pathol. 1989;42:800–4.
5. Koufman JA. The otolaryngologic manifestations of gastroesophageal reflux disease (GERD): a clinical investigation of 225 patients using ambulatory 24-hour pH monitoring and an experimental investigation of the role of acid and pepsin in the development of laryngeal injury. Laryngoscope. 1991;101:1–64.
6. Lechien JR, Bock JM, Carroll TL, Akst LM. Is empirical treatment a reasonable strategy for laryngopharyngeal reflux? A contemporary review. Clin Otolaryngol. 2020;45(4):450–8.
7. Santos PM, Afrassiabi A, Weymuller EA. Risk factors associated with prolonged intubation and laryngeal injury. Otolaryngol Head Neck Surg. 1994;111:453–c459.
8. Benjamin B, Roche J. Vocal granuloma, including sclerosis of the arytenoid cartilage: radiographic findings. Ann Otol Rhinol Laryngol. 1993;102:756–60.
9. Manolopoulos L, Stavroulaki P, Yiotakis J, et al. CO_2 and KTP-532 laser cordectomy for bilateral vocal fold paralysis. J Laryngol Otol. 1999;113:637–41.
10. Galli A, Giordano L, Sarandria D, Di Santo D, Bussi M. Oncological and complication assessment of CO2 laser-assisted endoscopic surgery for T1-T2 glottic tumours: clinical experience. Acta Otorhinolaryngol Ital. 2016;36(3):167–73.
11. Hoffman HT, Overholt E, Karnell M, McCulloch TM. Vocal process granuloma. Head Neck. 2001;23(12):1061–74.
12. Shumrick KA, Shumrick SA, Vietti M. Inflammatory diseases of the larynx. In: Fried MP, editor. The larynx a multidisciplinary approach. 2nd ed. St. Louis: Mosby; 1996. p. 283–307.
13. Ward PH, Zwitman D, Hanson D, Berci G. Contact ulcers and granulomas of the larynx: new insights into their etiology as a basis for more rational treatment. Otolaryngol Head Neck Surg. 1980;88:262–9.
14. New GB, Devine KD. Contact ulcer granuloma. Ann Otol Rhinol Laryngol. 1949;58:548–58.

15. Ding L, Lv T, Lou Z. The recurrent factors of idiopathic vocal process granulomas after cold steel excision. Am J Otolaryngol. 2022;43(3):103454.
16. Nasri S, Sercarz JA, McAlpin T, Berke GS. Treatment of vocal fold granuloma using botulinum toxin type A. Laryngoscope. 1995;105(6):585–8.
17. Pham Q, Campbell R, Mattioni J, Sataloff R. Botulinum toxin injections into the lateral cricoarytenoid muscles for vocal process granuloma. J Voice. 2018;32(3):363–6.
18. Hamdan AL, Khalifee E, Jaffal H, Ghanem A. Interarytenoid botulinum toxin A injection for the treatment of vocal process granuloma. J Laryngol Otol. 2019;133(12):1041–5.
19. Fink DS, Achkar J, Franco RA, Song PC. Interarytenoid botulinum toxin injection for recalcitrant vocal process granuloma. Laryngoscope. 2013;123(12):3084–7.
20. Ho CF, Lee YC, Hsin LJ, Lee LA, Li HY, Fang TJ. Low-dose LEMG-guided botulinum toxin type A injection for intractable vocal process granulomas. J Voice. 2022;36(2):277–82.
21. Damrose EJ, Damrose JF. Botulinum toxin as adjunctive therapy in refractory laryngeal granuloma. J Laryngol Otol. 2008;122(8):824–8.
22. Pan Y, Li J, Zhang J, Wang X, Jia Y. Thyroarytenoid botulinum toxin injection for refractory laryngeal contact granuloma. Am J Otolaryngol. 2022;43(4):103482.
23. Qiang Y, Liu XH, Zhang QQ, Xie M, Guo RX, Shi Y, Yang HN, Cao N, Luo HN. The effectiveness of various treatment approaches for laryngeal contact granulomas. Eur Arch Otorrinolaringol. 2024;281(4):1877–84.
24. Hamdan AL, Hosri J, Helou V, Mourad M. Transnasal endoscopic injection of botulinum toxin in patients with adductor spasmodic dysphonia. Iran J Otorhinolaryngol. 2024;36(5):595–601.
25. Ford CN, Bless DM, Patel NY. Botulinum toxin treatment of spasmodic dysphonia: techniques, indications, efficacy. J Voice. 1992;6(4):370–6.

9 Office-Based Steroid Injection Following Laser Therapy for Benign Lesions of the Vocal Folds

Despite the advances in technology and the use of more refined instruments, scar formation remains a feared complication of microlaryngeal surgery [1]. With scarring, there is a change in the lamina propria extracellular matrix—mainly, an increase in collagen and a decrease in elastin, among other constituents. This change in the extracellular matrix reduces the pliability of the vocal fold and increases its stiffness. Risk factors for fibrosis and/or scar formation following microlaryngeal surgery are older age (above 50 years), duration of hoarseness of more than 6 months, and/or a lesion attached to the vocal ligament [2, 3].

In an attempt to reduce the prevalence of vocal fold scars, steroid injections following surgery have been advocated as a complementary treatment modality. The rationale behind this therapy is to decrease scar formation, similar to what has been reported in dermatology and plastic surgery [4]. Two mechanisms have been suggested: one is the anti-inflammatory effect, and the other is the modulation of fibroblast activity, thereby decreasing the synthesis of collagen and other glycosaminoglycans [5–10]. In the vocal folds, steroid injections can help regulate the extracellular matrix metabolism of fibroblasts, thus reducing their proliferation and biosynthesis [11].

Using immunostaining on normal rat vocal fold tissue, Zhou et al. reported the presence of glucocorticoid receptors in the epithelium and capillaries. The authors also noted that these receptors are expressed by the vocal fold fibroblasts, whose proliferation decreased with the use of exogenous steroids [12]. In 1992, Bouchayer and Cornut were the first to describe the use of steroid injections toward the end of microlaryngeal surgery for vocal fold benign lesions and scars. Following the elevation of a microflap and removal of the submucosal mass, hydrocortisone is injected into the surgical bed. The authors reported improvement in voice quality, associated with an increase in vocal fold closure and malleability [13]. In 1995, Courey et al. reported their experience with steroid injection following the excision of benign lesions of the vocal folds using the endoscopic vocal fold microflap technique. The authors noted the return of mucosal waves in 18 out of 24 vocal folds.

A. L. Hamdan, *Atlas of Office-based Laryngeal Steroid Injection*,
https://doi.org/10.1007/978-3-032-05235-3_9

The improvement in stroboscopic examination was associated with a self-perceived improvement in voice quality in the majority of patients [1]. In 2023, Cho et al. investigated the efficacy of steroid injections following microlaryngeal surgery for benign lesions of the vocal folds in a cohort of 211 patients and noted a significantly lower risk of persistent dysphonia in the subgroup who had intralesional injections combined with microlaryngeal surgery, compared to those who had only microlaryngeal surgery. Moreover, those who had adjuvant intralesional steroid injections had a significantly lower recurrence rate than those who did not [2].

These clinical reports are in agreement with numerous histomorphometric and histologic studies asserting the positive effect of steroid injection on healing following elevation of a mucosal flap. Coleman et al conducted a histomorphometric and functional study on the impact of corticosteroids on the healing of vocal fold lateral microflaps, and showed a delay in the inflammatory and neovascular responses at 12 and 21 days, respectively. The study was conducted on 15 dogs, where one vocal fold was treated with steroids and the other was used as a control [14]. Campagnolo et al evaluated the effect of dexamethasone sodium phosphate infiltration on wound healing of vocal fold rabbits and found a significant reduction in collagen deposition 3 and 7 days after the injection.

The authors recommended the use of steroid injections in phonosurgery to prevent scar formation [15]. In an animal study using a rabbit model, Jeong et al. investigated the effect of steroid injection following KTP-laser-induced vocal fold scarring and noted a significant difference in vocal fold maximum amplitude vibration compared to controls. Histologic examination revealed a significant reduction in collagen density, and PCR analysis revealed an increase in Has-2 and Mmp-9 in the rabbit treated with steroids. The authors concluded that intralesional steroid injection helps mitigate vocal fold scarring in a rabbit model [16]. These findings encouraged the use of steroids as adjuvant therapy following surgical excision of benign lesions of the vocal folds.

The last two decades witnessed a reform in laryngology practice toward office-based surgery. Different treatment options under local anesthesia are offered to patients with benign lesions of the vocal folds, among which is laser therapy. Numerous reports confirmed that in-office laser therapy is successful in improving subjective and objective voice outcome measures.

Hamdan et al. conducted a systematic review and meta-analysis on the efficacy of office-based laser therapy for Reinke's edema. The authors reported significant improvement in the VHI-10 score and jitter, and significant disease regression. The review included 6 studies and 58 patients [17]. Abi Zeid Daou et al. conducted a similar review on the efficacy of office-based laser therapy for vocal fold polyps and reported a significant decrease in the mean VHI-10 score, GRB ratings, and a significant increase in maximum phonation time (MPT). The systematic review and meta-analysis included 10 studies and 242 participants [18]. Despite the well-established efficacy of office-based laser therapy, scar formation secondary to inadvertent heat injury to the deep structures of the vocal fold remains a feared complication.

Other potential complications include partial disease regression and recurrence of the lesion. The added value of steroid injection following office-based laser therapy has scarcely been investigated in the literature, despite the well-established benefit of its use in microlaryngeal surgery. In a study that included 42 patients who underwent office-based laser therapy, Hamdan et al. reported a significant difference in complete disease regression between those who underwent laser therapy and steroid injection versus those who underwent laser therapy alone (77.7% vs. 42.1%, respectively). Similarly, there was a significant difference in the decrease in the mean VHI-10 score between the two subgroups (-17.3 ± 11.8 vs. -10.5 ± 6.9, respectively) [19]. Future studies on larger cohorts are needed to establish the added value of steroid injections following office-based laser therapy.

9.1 Case 1

A 48-year-old, heavy smoker, presented to Voice clinic with hoarseness of a few months' duration. The patient denied any history of voice abuse, allergy, or reflux disease. His VHI-10 score at presentation was 7. Acoustic analysis revealed a fundamental frequency (F0) of 105.93 Hz, habitual pitch (HP) of 87.09 Hz, jitter of 0.28, shimmer of 1.59, noise-to-harmonics ratio (NHR) of 0.123, and voice turbulence index (VTI) of 0.028. His maximum phonation time (MPT) was 15.65 s. Laryngeal flexible endoscopic examination revealed a non-hemorrhagic polyp on the anterior one-third of the left vocal fold and a reactive lesion opposite to the side.

The patient underwent office-based blue laser therapy for the left vocal fold polyp using the contact and non-contact modes (Fig. 9.1a, b). Following the laser therapy, 1.5 cc of dexamethasone (8 mg/2 ml) was injected into the surgical bed using a 25-gauge flexible needle (Fig. 9.1c). The procedure was tolerated well by the patient, with no complications noted.

On follow-up 3 weeks later, the patient had significant improvement in his voice quality, with a drop in his VHI-10 score to 1. Acoustic analysis revealed an increase in the F0 to 111.81, HP to 94.17 Hz. There was also an increase in MPT to 17.49 s. Laryngeal examination revealed almost complete regression of the polyp with mild edema and redness at the surgical bed (Fig. 9.1d).

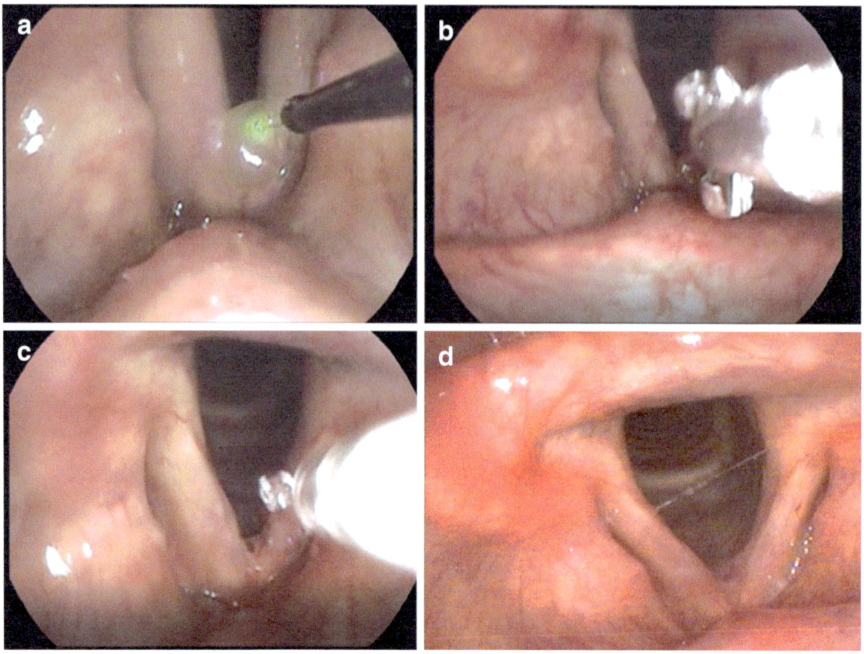

Fig. 9.1 (**a**) An endoscopic view of the larynx showing the blue laser glass fiber in contact with the left vocal fold polyp. (**b**) An endoscopic view showing the cup-forceps directed toward the left vocal fold lesion. (**c**) An endoscopic view showing the 25-gauge needle directed toward the surgical bed following the blue laser therapy. A total of 0.1 cc of Dexamethasone (8 mg/2 ml) was injected. (**d**) An endoscopic view of the larynx showing almost complete regression of the lesion. Note the presence of mild edema and redness along the lower lip of the left vocal fold

9.2 Case 2

A 45-year-old man, a heavy smoker, presented to the Voice Clinic with hoarseness of 2 weeks duration. The patient had a history of voice abuse and denied any history of allergy or reflux disease. His VHI-10 score was 26. Acoustic analysis revealed a fundamental frequency (F0) of 119.48 Hz, habitual pitch (HP) 115.05 Hz, jitter of 1.04, shimmer of 3.39, noise-to-harmonics ratio (NHR) of 0.101, and voice turbulence index (VTI) of 0.055. His maximum phonation time (MPT) was 11.52 s. Laryngeal flexible endoscopic evaluation showed a non-hemorrhagic polyp on the right vocal fold and a reactive lesion on the left vocal fold.

The patient underwent office-based blue laser therapy for the right vocal fold polyp using contact and non-contact modes (Fig. 9.2a). Following the laser therapy, 0.2 cc of dexamethasone (8 mg/2 ml) was injected in the right vocal fold, and 0.1 cc was injected into the reactive lesion on the left using the transnasal approach (Fig. 9.2b). The procedure was tolerated well by the patient with no complications noted.

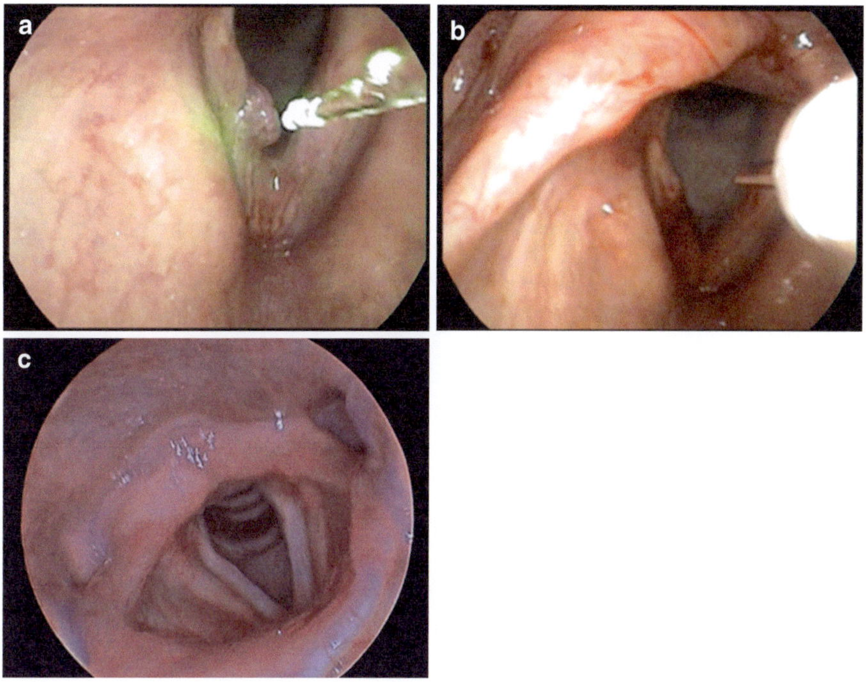

Fig. 9.2 (**a**) An endoscopic view showing the blue laser glass fiber (400 μm) directed toward the right vocal fold polyp. (**b**) An endoscopic view showing a 25-gauge needle directed toward the surgical bed following the blue laser therapy of the right vocal fold polyp. A total of 0.2 cc of dexamethasone (8 mg/2 ml) was injected. (**c**) An endoscopic view of the larynx showing complete regression of the right vocal fold polyp

On follow-up 6 weeks later, the patient had a significant improvement in his voice quality, with a drop in his VHI-10 score to 1. Acoustic analysis revealed a decrease in jitter of 0.726 and shimmer of 2.98, and an increase in MPT of 22.38 s. Laryngeal examination revealed complete regression of the polyp (Fig. 9.2c).

9.3 Case 3

A 48-year-old man presented with a history of hoarseness of 4 weeks' duration following voice abuse. The patient had no history of smoking, allergy, or reflux disease. Auditory-perceptual evaluation revealed grade 2 dysphonia. His Voice Handicap Index-10 (VHI-10) score was 6. Acoustic analysis showed a habitual pitch of 137.2 Hz, jitter of 1.07, shimmer of 2.62, noise-to-harmonics ratio (NHR) of 0.07, voice turbulence index (VTI) of 0.045, and maximum phonation time (MPT) of 19.03 s. Laryngeal flexible endoscopic examination revealed a hemorrhagic polyp with a feeding vessel at the anterior one-third of the left vocal fold. A reactive lesion was noted on the right vocal fold.

The patient underwent office-based thulium laser therapy for the left vocal fold polyp using the contact and non-contact modes. The laser setting used was power 3 W, pulse mode frequency 2 Hz, aiming beam 65% (Fig. 9.3a–c). Following the laser therapy, a 25-gauge needle was introduced percutaneously through the thyrohyoid membrane and directed toward the surgical bed. A 0.1–0.2 cc of

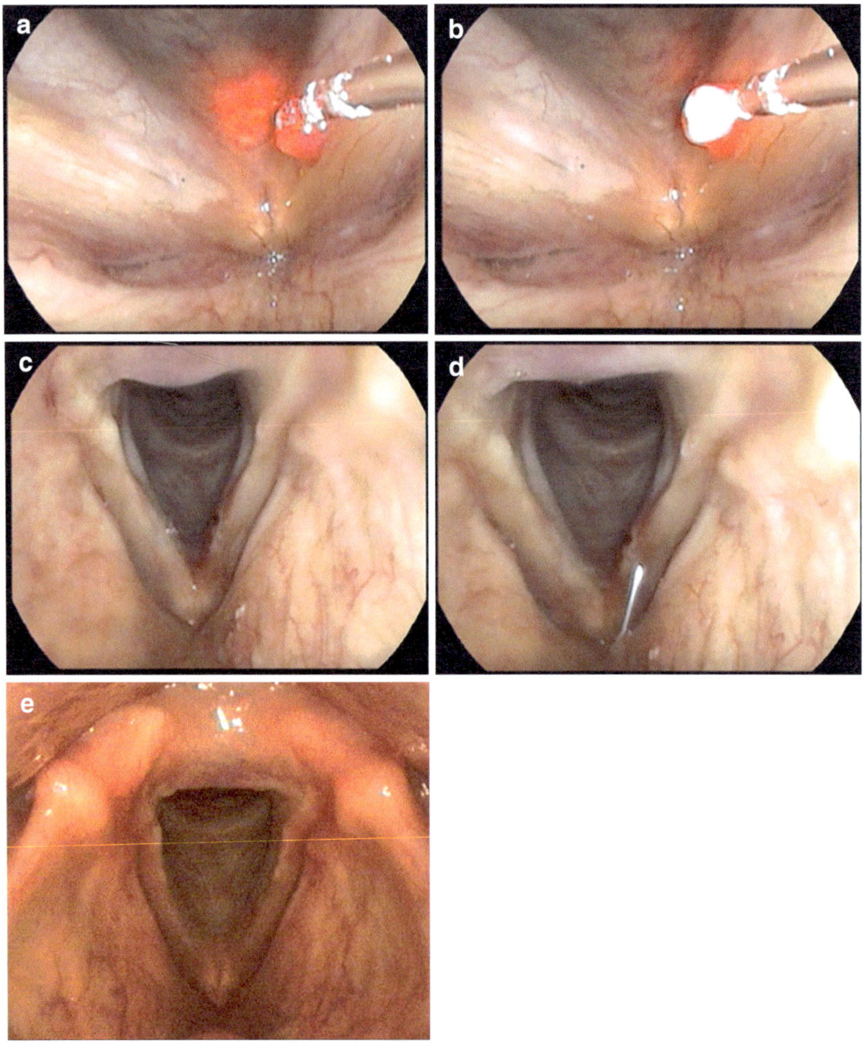

Fig. 9.3 (**a**) An endoscopic view during surgery showing the thulium laser beam directed toward the polyp in a non-contact mode. (**b**) An endoscopic view of the larynx intra-operatively showing blanching of the lesion following application of the laser beam. (**c**) An endoscopic view of the larynx showing end-point surgery. (**d**) An endoscopic view showing the tip of a 25-gauge needle inserted submucosally before injecting 0.1–0.2 cc dexamethasone (1 mg/ml). (**e**) An endoscopic view of the larynx 7 weeks after surgery showing complete regression of the lesion with minimal hyperemia at the surgical bed

dexamethasone (4 ml/1 mg) was injected submucosally at the base of the lesion (Fig. 9.3d). The procedure was tolerated well by the patient, with no complications noted.

On follow-up 7 weeks later, the patient had marked improvement in his voice quality with a drop in his VHI-10 score to 3. Auditory perceptual evaluation revealed a normal voice. Acoustic analysis showed a decrease in habitual pitch to 113.5 Hz, a decrease in jitter of 0.46, and an increase in maximum phonation time to 22.3 s. Laryngeal examination showed complete regression of the polyp (Fig. 9.3e).

9.4 Case 4

A 38-year-old man presented with dysphonia of a few weeks' duration. He had a positive history of smoking and phonotrauma. His VHI-10 score at presentation was 19. Auditory perceptual evaluation revealed grade 3 dysphonia, Laryngeal examination using the flexible nasopharyngoscope revealed a hemorrhagic polyp at the anterior one-third of the left vocal fold (Fig. 9.4a).

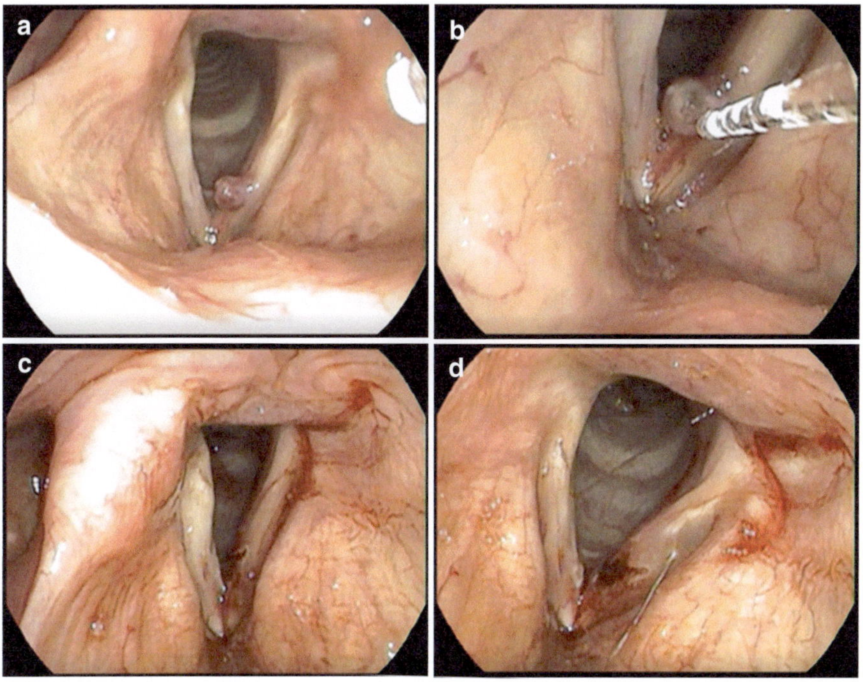

Fig. 9.4 (**a**) An endoscopic view of the larynx showing a left vocal fold hemorrhagic polyp occupying almost the entire anterior one-third. (**b**) An endoscopic view of the larynx showing the thulium laser glass fiber (550 μm) aiming at the lesion. Note the blanching of the polyp due to the thermal effect of the laser. (**c**) An endoscopic view of the larynx showing complete disappearance of the lesion. Note mild charring at the surgical bed. (**d**) An endoscopic view showing the tip of a 25-gauge needle inserted submucosally into the left vocal fold for the injection of 0.1 cc of dexamethasone (4 m/ml). The thyrohyoid approach was used for the introduction of the needle

The patient underwent office-based thulium laser therapy for the left vocal fold polyp, followed by dexamethasone injection (0.1 cc of 4 mg/ml solution) at the surgical bed using the thyrohyoid approach (Fig. 9.4b–d).

9.5 Case 5

A 63-year-old female patient presented to the Voice Unit with hoarseness following voice abuse a few months before her presentation. Auditory perceptual evaluation revealed grade 2 dysphonia. Her VHI-10 score was 22. Laryngeal examination showed a gelatinous polyp at the mid-membranous portion of the left vocal fold.

The patient underwent office-based thulium laser therapy for the left vocal fold polyp using a 550 μm glass fiber at power 3, pulsed mode with frequency 2 Hz (Fig. 9.5a–c). The laser therapy was followed by the injection of 0.2 cc of dexamethasone (4 mg/ml) at the surgical bed using the transnasal approach (Fig. 9.5d).

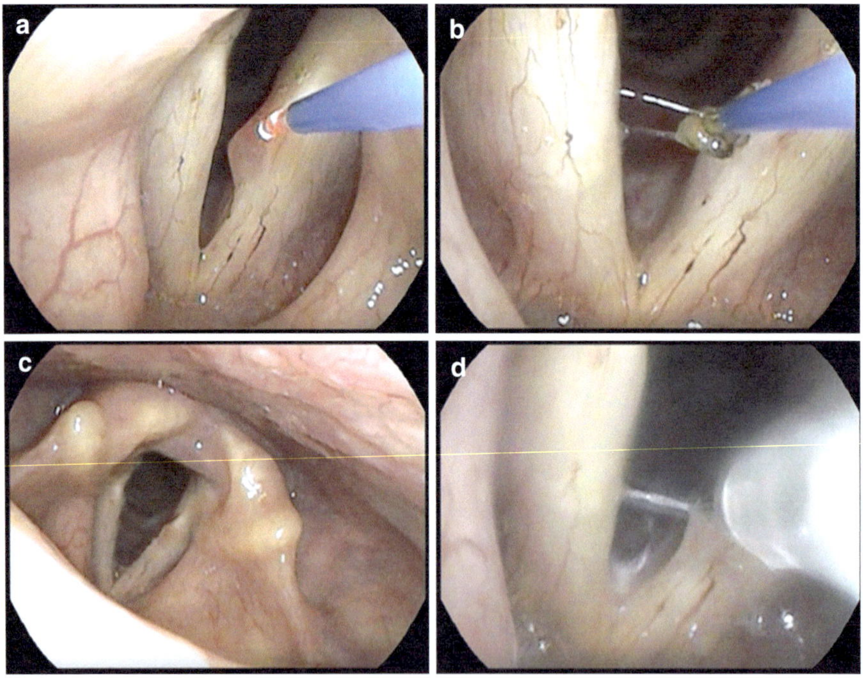

Fig. 9.5 (**a**) An endoscopic view of the larynx showing the thulium laser beam directed to the site of the polyp. (**b**) An endoscopic view showing the tip of the glass fiber used to remove the gelatinous content of the polypoid lesion. (**c**) An endoscopic view showing the endpoint of laser application. (**d**) An endoscopic view of the larynx showing the tip of the 25-gauge flexible needle directed toward the surgical bed following laser therapy

9.6 Case 6

A 29-year-old male presented to the Voice Clinic with a few months' history of hoarseness. The patient was a smoker but he denied any history of reflux disease or allergy. His Voice Handicap Index-10 (VHI-10) score at presentation was 26. On perceptual evaluation, he had grade 2 dysphonia. Acoustic analysis showed a fundamental frequency (F_0) of 137.02 Hz, habitual pitch (HP) of 152.8 Hz, jitter of 3.24, shimmer of 12.61, noise-to-harmonics ratio (NHR) of 0.151, and voice turbulence index (VTI) of 0.093. His maximum phonation time (MPT) was 6.52 s. On laryngeal examination, he had a right anterior vocal fold polyp with a reactive lesion on the opposite side (Fig. 9.6a).

The patient underwent in-office blue laser therapy for his vocal fold polyp using non-contact and contact modes (Fig. 9.6b, c). Following laser therapy, 0.35 cc of dexamethasone (8 mg/2 mL) was injected submucosally in the right vocal fold and 0.2 cc in the left vocal fold (Fig. 9.6d).

On follow-up 6 weeks later, the patient had marked improvement in his voice quality.

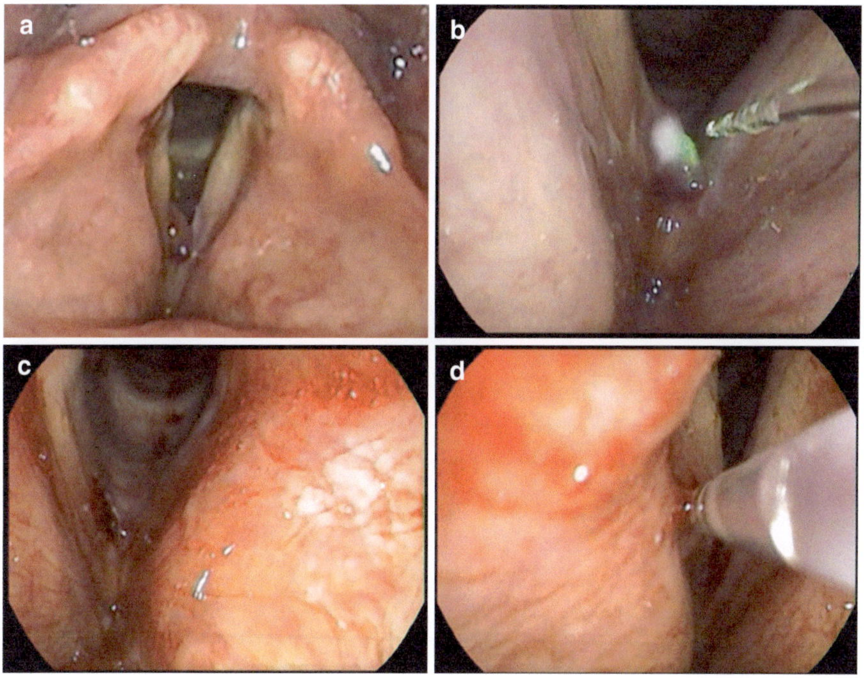

Fig. 9.6 (**a**) An endoscopic view of the larynx showing a right vocal fold hemorrhagic polyp. (**b**) An intraoperative view showing blanching of the right vocal fold polyp during the blue laser therapy. (**c**) A view of the larynx toward the end of the laser session. Note the complete disappearance of the lesion. (**d**) An intraoperative view showing steroid injection at the surgical bed following the laser therapy

9.7 Case 7

A 45-year-old male presented to the Voice Clinic with a few weeks' history of hoarseness following voice abuse. The patient was an occasional smoker and denied any history of reflux disease or allergy. His Voice Handicap Index-10 score (VHI-10) at presentation was 27. On perceptual evaluation, he exhibited grade 2 dysphonia, grade 2 roughness, grade 1 breathiness, grade 0 asthenia and grade 0 strain. Acoustic analysis showed a fundamental frequency (F0) of 129.28 Hz, habitual pitch (HP) of 121.84 Hz, jitter of 1.17, shimmer of 4.89, noise-to-harmonics ratio (NHR) of 0.155, and voice turbulence index (VTI) of 0.068. His maximum phonation time (MPT) was 10 s. On laryngeal examination, he was found to have a left vocal fold polyp (Fig. 9.7a).

The patient underwent in-office blue laser therapy using non-contact and contact modes. Then, he was injected with 0.2 cc of dexamethasone (8 mg/2 ml) in both vocal folds (Fig. 9.7b).

Follow-up examination 6 weeks later showed complete disease regression with persistent redness and edema at the site of surgery.

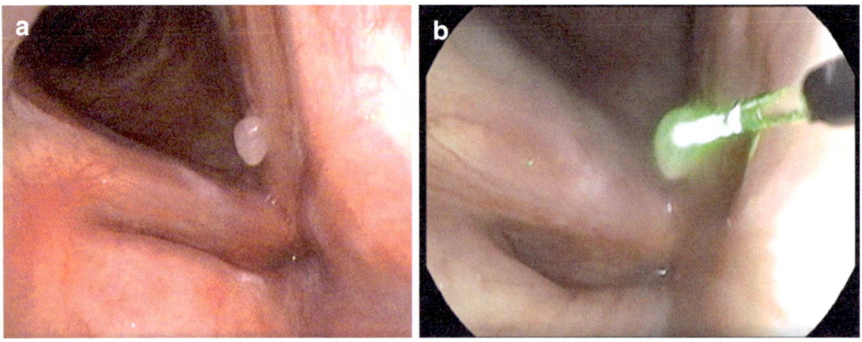

Fig. 9.7 (**a**) An endoscopic view of the larynx showing a left vocal fold gelatinous polyp. (**b**) An image showing the blue laser in non-contact mode during the treatment of a left vocal fold gelatinous polyp

9.8 Case 8

A 58-year-old man presented to the voice clinic with hoarseness of a few months' duration. The patient had a positive history of smoking and denied any history of allergy, reflux disease, or voice abuse. His Voice Handicap Index-10 (VHI-10) score was 5. Acoustic analysis revealed a fundamental frequency (F0) of 99.73 Hz, habitual pitch (HP) of 91.87 Hz, jitter of 0.498, shimmer of 2.18, noise-to-harmonics ratio (NHR) of 0.125, and voice turbulence index (VTI) of 0.027. His maximum phonation time (MPT) was 4.75 s. Laryngeal endoscopic evaluation revealed bilateral vocal fold edema and a right vocal fold polypoid lesion (Fig. 9.8a).

The patient underwent office-based blue laser therapy for both lesions using the contact and non-contact modes. Following laser therapy, dexamethasone (8 mg/2 ml) was injected into both vocal folds. The procedure was tolerated well by the patient with no complications noted (Fig. 9.8b).

On follow-up 6 weeks later, the patient reported improvement in his voice quality. His VHI-10 score dropped to 1. There were no significant changes in acoustic and aerodynamic parameters. Laryngeal examination revealed almost complete disease regression (Fig. 9.8c).

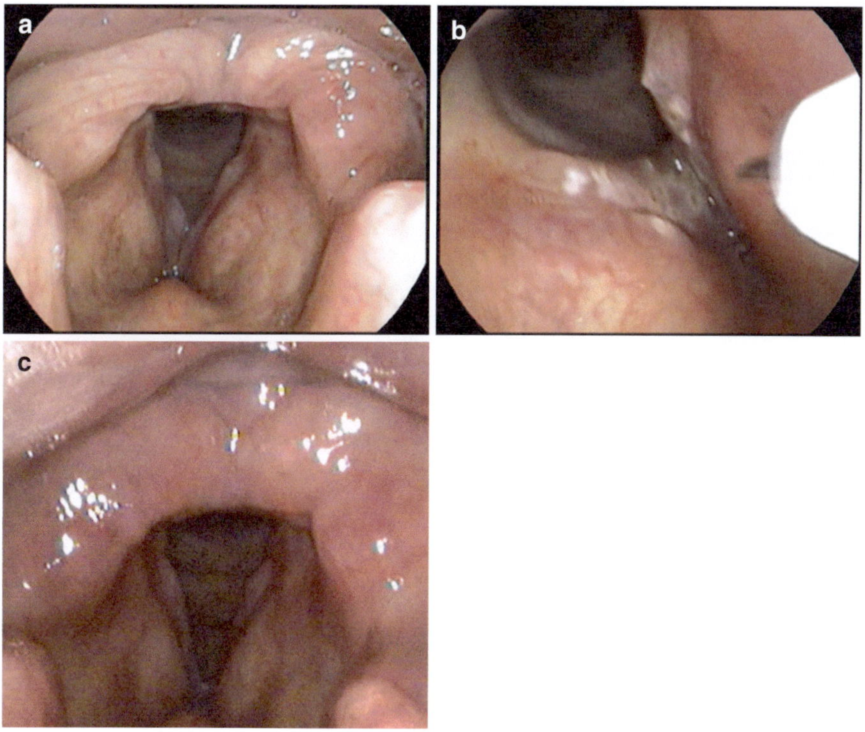

Fig. 9.8 (**a**) An endoscopic view of the larynx showing bilateral vocal fold edema and a left vocal fold polypoid lesion. (**b**) An intraoperative view showing blanching at the site of blue laser therapy. Note the tip of the needle directed toward the surgical bed. (**c**) An endoscopic view of the larynx 6 weeks after surgery showing marked disease regression

References

1. Courey MS, Stone RE, Gardner GM, Ossoff RH. Endoscopic vocal fold microflap: a three-year experience. Ann Otol Rhinol Laryngol. 1995;104(4):267–73.
2. Cho JH, Kim SY, Joo YH, et al. Efficacy and safety of adjunctive steroid injection after microsurgical removal of benign vocal fold lesions. J Voice. 2017;31(5):615–20.
3. Wu PH, Wang CT. Risk factors for postoperative vocal fold fibrosis following microlaryngeal surgery. Laryngoscope Investig Otolaryngol. 2023;8(5):1324–7.
4. Chowdri NA, Mattoo MM, Darzi MA. Keloids and hypertrophic scars: results with intra-operative and serial postoperative corticosteroid injection therapy. Aust N Z J Surg. 1999;69(9):655–9.
5. Sherris DA, Larrabee WF, Murakami CS. Management of scar contractures, hypertrophic scars, and keloids. Otolaryngol Clin N Am. 1995;28:1057–68.
6. Gadson PF, Russell JD, Russell SB. Glucocorticoid receptors in human fibroblasts derived from normal dermis and keloid tissue. J Biol Chem. 1984;259:11236–41.
7. Krusche T, Worret WI. Mechanical properties of keloids in vivo during treatment with intralesional triamcinolone acetonide. Arch Dermatol Res. 1995;287:289–93.
8. McCoy BJ, Diegelmann RF, Cohen IK. In vitro inhibition of cell growth collagen synthesis, and prolyl hydroxylase activity by triamcinolone acetonide. Proc Soc Exp Biol Med. 1980;163:216–22.
9. Kauh YC, Rouda S, Mondragon G, et al. Major suppression of pro-alpha1(I) type I collagen gene expression in the dermis after keloid excision and immediate intrawound injection of triamcinolone acetonide. J Am Acad Dermatol. 1997;37:586–9.
10. Lavker RM, Schechter NM. Cutaneous mast cell depletion results from topical corticosteroid usage. J Immunol. 1985;135:2368–73.
11. Tang YW. Intra- and postoperative steroid injections for keloids and hypertrophic scars. Br J Plast Surg. 1992;45(5):371–3.
12. Zhou H, Sivasankar M, Kraus DH, Sandulache VC, Amin M, Branski RC. Glucocorticoids regulate extracellular matrix metabolism in human vocal fold fibroblasts. Laryngoscope. 2011;121(9):1915–9.
13. Bouchayer M, Cornut G. Microsurgical treatment of benign vocal fold lesions: indications, technique, results. Folia Phoniatr Logop. 1992;44(3–4):155–84.
14. Coleman JR Jr, Smith S, Reinisch L, et al. Histomorphometric and laryngeal videostroboscopic analysis of the effects of corticosteroids on microflap healing in the dog larynx. Ann Otol Rhinol Laryngol. 1999;108(2):119–27.
15. Campagnolo AM, Tsuji DH, Sennes LU, et al. Histologic study of acute vocal fold wound healing after corticosteroid injection in a rabbit model. Ann Otol Rhinol Laryngol. 2010;119(2):133–9.
16. Jeong JY, Thapa S, Lee SW. Does intralesional steroid injection effectively mitigate vocal fold scarring in a rabbit model? Laryngoscope. 2025;135(1):176–82.
17. Hamdan AL, Abi Zeid Daou C, Ghanem A, A R Feghali P, Hosri J, Sataloff RT. Office-based laser therapy in reinke's edema: a systematic review and meta-analysis. J Voice. 2025;39(3):799–805. https://doi.org/10.1016/j.jvoice.2022.12.003. Epub 2023 Jan 19. PMID: 36681567.
18. Abi Zeid Daou C, Ghanem A, Hosri J, Abou Raji Feghali P, Hamdan AL. Office-based laser therapy in vocal fold polyps: a systematic review and meta-analysis. J Voice. 2023;S0892–1997(23)00095-4. https://doi.org/10.1016/j.jvoice.2023.03.003. Epub ahead of print. PMID: 37003865.
19. Hamdan AL, Ghanem A, Abi Zeid Daou C, Hosri J, Feghali PAR, Jabbour C, Alam E. The added value of steroid injection following office-based blue laser therapy of benign lesions of the vocal folds; short-term effect in a cohort of 43 patients. J Voice. 2025;39(4):934–39. https://doi.org/10.1016/j.jvoice.2023.02.012. Epub 2023 Mar 15. PMID: 36925408.

10 Office-Based Steroid Injection for Bamboo Nodes and Mucosal Tear

10.1 Office-Based Steroid Injection for Vocal Fold Bamboo Nodes

Autoimmune diseases can affect all components of the phonatory system including the larynx. There is growing evidence in the literature suggesting an increase in the prevalence of voice and swallowing disorders in patients with autoimmune disorders. It is estimated that two out of three patients may present with a change in voice quality or vocal fatigue [1]. This is not surprising given that the larynx, similar to other musculoskeletal structures in the body, consists of muscles and diarthrodial joints.

The voice and swallowing symptoms in patients with autoimmune diseases vary with the severity and stage of the disease. In the acute phase, patients present with neck pain, dysphagia, hoarseness, globus sensation, and referred otalgia whereas, in chronic cases patients may present with airway symptoms such as shortness of breath and respiratory discomfort. Suggested mechanisms for laryngeal involvement include chronic inflammation, deposition of immune complexes, and recurrent laryngeal nerve dysfunction as a result of mass compression [2, 3].

The most common laryngeal findings on examination are edema and erythema of the mucosal lining, and dryness of the vocal folds, suggestive of sicca laryngitis [4]. The repeated remission and exacerbation of the autoimmune disease may also lead to structural deformities in the larynx with bone destruction and joint deformities [5]. Patients may also present with impaired mobility or fixation of one or both vocal folds. The impairment in mobility can be mechanical secondary to the involvement of the cricoarytenoid (CAJ) joint by the autoimmune disease or neurogenic

---

Supplementary Information The online version contains supplementary material available at https://doi.org/10.1007/978-3-032-05235-3_10.

A. L. Hamdan, *Atlas of Office-based Laryngeal Steroid Injection*,
https://doi.org/10.1007/978-3-032-05235-3_10

secondary to vasculitis or thrombosis to the vasa nervosa of the recurrent laryngeal nerves [6]. Radiologic imaging using high-resolution computerized tomography may reveal CAJ abnormalities such as narrowing, ankylosis, erosion, and increased soft tissue densities in 72% of the cases [7].

Other rare laryngeal findings on examination include impaired mobility of the vocal folds, rheumatoid nodules and bamboo nodes (Fig. 10.1). Bamboo nodes were initially described by Hosako et al. in 1993 in reference to a yellowish submucosal lesion fusiform in shape located at a perpendicular axis to the vocal fold. On histologic examination, the lesion had central necrosis surrounded by inflammatory cells [8]. Bamboo nodes have rarely been reported in the literature since their initial description. In 2001, Perouse et al. reported 19 patients with transverse yellowish lesions of the vocal folds that were treated surgically via a cordotomy. Eight out of the 19 patients had a history of autoimmune disorders [9]. In 2001, Murano et al. reported two patients with no pre-existing autoimmune diseases who presented with hoarseness and vocal folds bamboo nodes on laryngeal examination. After thorough investigation, one patient was diagnosed with Sjögren's syndrome, and the second one with Systemic Lupus Erythematosus [10].

In 2007, Schwemmie and Ptok reported a 43-year-old woman diagnosed with Sharp syndrome who complained of dysphonia that was attributed to a bamboo node on the vocal fold. The authors noted that a change in voice quality may be the presenting symptom of patients with autoimmune diseases, and the need for otolaryngologists to familiarize themselves with this rare pathologic finding on laryngeal examination [11].

In 2018, Todic et al. reviewed the demographic characteristics and treatment of ten patients diagnosed with bamboo nodes on laryngeal examination and noted that all patients were women, and all had a history of autoimmune disease except for one. The management consisted of one or more of the following modalities: speech therapy, oral steroids, surgery, and laryngeal steroid injections. The authors again reiterated the need for a high index of suspicion to diagnose these lesions in patients at risk [12].

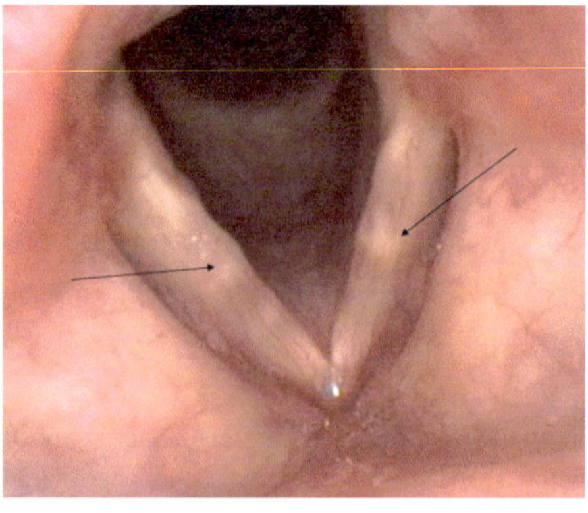

Fig. 10.1 A female patient with a history of Hashimoto's disease presented with progressive hoarseness. Flexible laryngoscopy showed bilateral vocal fold bamboo nodes. Note that these yellowish lesions are submucosal and perpendicular to the long axis of the vocal fold

In 2021, Lagos et al. reported six patients with underlying autoimmune diseases who presented with dysphonia. Laryngeal vide-stroboscopic examination revealed bamboo nodes in all cases and impaired mucosal waves in four of them. Patients were treated conservatively with speech therapy, and control of reflux and were referred for immunosuppressive therapy. Most patients had marked improvement in auditory perceptual evaluation following treatment. The authors stressed the need for a rheumatologic work-up in patients with dysphonia and bamboo nodes [13].

10.2 Vocal Fold Mucosal Tear

Dysphonia is defined as a change in voice quality in relation to pitch, loudness, or timbre [14]. Common causes include structural disorders such as polyps, nodules, and cysts, neurologic disorders such as vocal fold paralysis, and functional voice disorders such as muscle tension dysphonia [15]. A rare condition that may lead to dysphonia and that is often missed is vocal fold mucosal tear (Fig. 10.2).

The first case report of vocal fold mucosal tear and hemorrhage was reported by Sataloff et al. in 1994 [16]. In 2001, Hoover et al. described the clinical presentation and treatment of four additional cases. The authors stressed the need to consider this entity in the differential diagnosis of dysphonia in singers [17]. The main predisposing factor for vocal fold mucosal tear is phonotrauma. Because of their high vocal demand, professional voice users are at a higher risk than non-professional voice users. Phonotrauma may be in the form of a cough or repetitive throat clearing, which leads to an increase in the collision force between the vocal folds.

Affected patients present with an array of symptoms such as inability to speak loudly, volume disturbance and feeling of mucus on the vocal folds. Singers may complain of tightness in the voice, loss of the high notes, loss of the low register, or "singing on a brittle cords" as reported by Sataloff et al. in their publication on mucosal tears in singers [16].

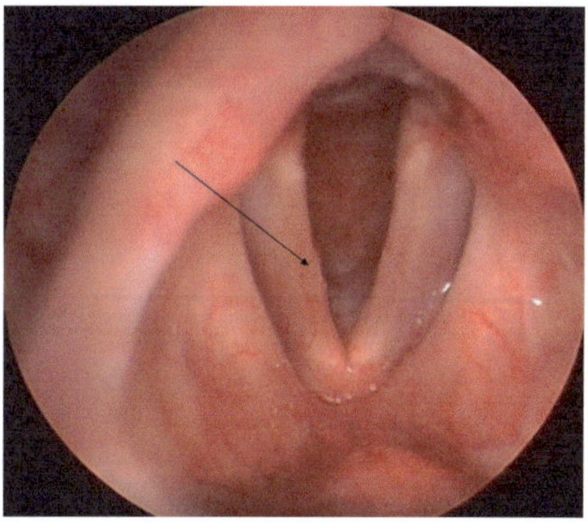

Fig. 10.2 A 53-year-old man, a singer, presented with a history of hoarseness following a vocal performance. On laryngeal examination, he had a right vocal fold mucosal tear. The patient was advised voice rest, and a short course of steroids

On laryngeal examination, a high index of suspicion is needed in order not to miss the diagnosis. Hoover et al. highlighted the subtle findings on endoscopy, which can be easily missed or underdiagnosed [17]. Stroboscopy can show irregularity on the free edge of the vocal fold and or the presence of a white patch on the vibratory margin.

The treatment of mucosal tears of the vocal fold is conservative. Voice rest and the administration of anti-inflammatory agents are often recommended. In case of a concomitant airway infection, antibiotics may be prescribed to control the infectious process. If left untreated, or in case of no response to treatment, vocal fold scar may ensue, necessitating intralesional steroid injection.

10.3 Case 1

A young female patient, a non-smoker, presented with a history of a change in voice quality that was progressive over the last few years. The patient denied any history of voice abuse or overuse. Her medical history was positive for an autoimmune disease. Laryngeal examination showed bilateral, submucosal vocal fold yellowish masses consistent with bamboo nodes.

The patient underwent office-based intralesional steroid injections under local anesthesia. Using the thyrohyoid approach, 0.1 cc of triamcinolone acetonide (40 mg/ml) was injected submucosally at the lesion (Fig. 10.3a, Video 10.1).

On follow-up 6 weeks later, the patient had marked improvement in voice quality, and partial disease regression (Fig. 10.3b).

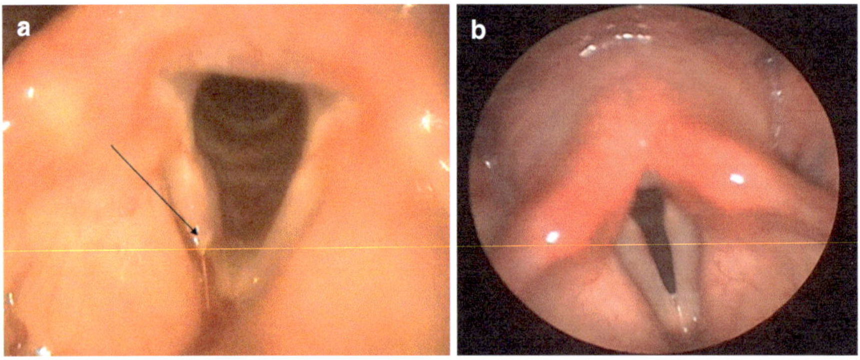

Fig. 10.3 (**a**) An endoscopic view of the larynx showing a 25-gauge needle inserted into the right vocal fold within the bamboo node. A 0.1 cc of triamcinolone acetonide was injected submucosally. (**b**) An endoscopic view of the larynx 3 months later showing almost complete disease regression

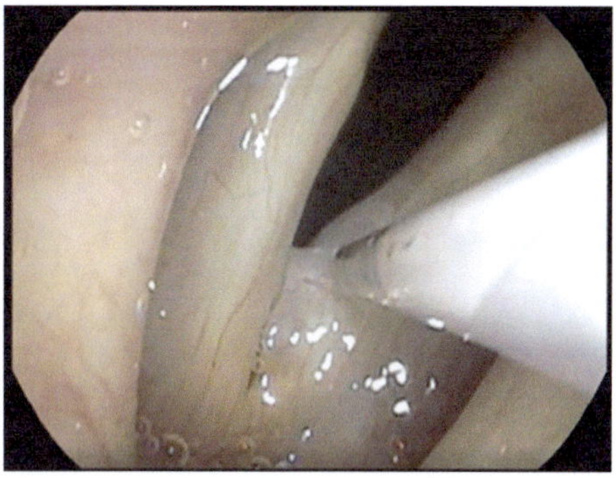

Fig. 10.4 An endoscopic view of the larynx showing a bleb formation following the injection of 0.1–0.2 cc dexamethasone into the left vocal fold

10.4 Case 2

A 50-year-old man, non-smoker, presented with a history of acute dysphonia that started following voice abuse. The patient had a negative medical history. On laryngeal examination, he had a left vocal fold mucosal tear. The patient was advised voice rest for 3–5 days.

On follow-up 6 weeks later, he had persistent changes in voice quality, and laryngeal examination showed mucosal thickening at the free edge of the left vocal fold. The patient was advised intralesional steroid injection. Under local anesthesia, 0.1–0.2 cc of dexamethasone (8 mg/2 ml) was injected submucosally at the site of injury (Fig. 10.4). The procedure was tolerated well by the patient, and no complications were noted.

10.5 Case 3

A 49-year-old man presented to the voice clinic with hoarseness of a few months' duration. The patient denied a history of smoking, voice abuse, and reflux disease. Laryngeal examination showed bilateral swelling of the vocal folds and a right vocal fold biofilm, all suggestive of a non-specific chronic inflammation. He was initially prescribed a course of Fluconazole 150 mg/day for 10 days and two courses of antibiotics to no avail. The patient underwent an office-based biopsy of the right vocal fold biofilm, which revealed squamous epithelium with reactive changes.

This was followed by office-based intralesional steroid injection using a 25-gauge flexible needle via the transnasal approach. A total of 0.25 cc of dexamethasone (8 mg/2 ml) was injected into each vocal fold (Fig. 10.5). The procedure was tolerated well by the patient with no complications noted. On follow-up 2 weeks later, the patient reported improvement in voice quality.

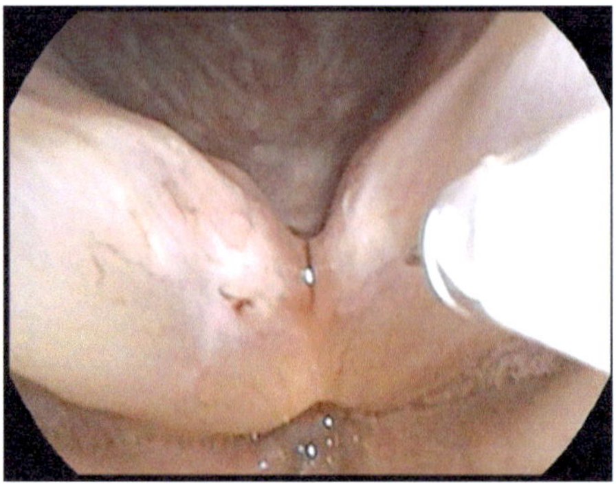

Fig. 10.5 An endoscopic view of the larynx following the bilateral intralesional steroid injection

10.6 Case 4

A 31-year-old man, non-smoker, presented to the voice clinic with a history of hoarseness and intermittent neck pain. The patient had a positive history of reflux disease. There was no history of voice abuse. His Voice Handicap Index-10 (VHI-10) score was 0. Acoustic analysis showed a fundamental frequency (F0) of 102.91 Hz, habitual pitch (HP) of 92.92 Hz, jitter of 0.352, shimmer of 1.535, noise-to-harmonics ratio (NHR) of 0.130, and voice turbulence index (VTI) of 0.035. Her maximum phonation time (MPT) was 27.77 s. Laryngeal flexible endoscopic evaluation revealed bilateral edema of the vocal folds, a lesion on the right vocal fold, and a reactive lesion on the opposite side (Fig. 10.6a). The patient was advised vocal hygiene therapy and office-based intralesional steroid injection.

The patient underwent office-based intralesional steroid injection using a 25-gauge flexible needle that was introduced into the working channel of a flexible nasopharyngoscope. A total of 0.2 cc of dexamethasone was injected into each vocal fold. The procedure was tolerated well by the patient with no complications noted (Fig. 10.6b).

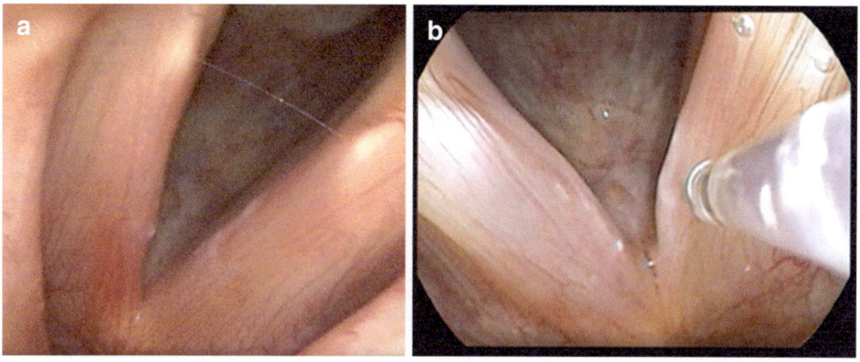

Fig. 10.6 (**a**) Laryngeal examination showing localized edema at the free edge of both vocal folds with a whitish lesion on the right vocal fold. (**b**) An endoscopic view of the larynx showing intralesional steroid injection using a flexible 25-gauge needle

10.7 Case 5

A 63-year-old man presented to the voice clinic with hoarseness and intermittent cough of a few months' duration. The patient was treated with antibiotics to no avail. He had a positive history of smoking. He denied any history of reflux disease, allergy, and phonotrauma. Endoscopic laryngeal examination revealed a leukoplakia on the free edge of the left vocal fold. Edema of both vocal folds was noted, with hyperemia more on the left side, suggestive of chronic inflammatory changes (Fig. 10.7a). The patient was prescribed a course of antibiotics and a steroid inhaler, following which there was no improvement.

The patient underwent office-based intralesional steroid injection using the 25-gauge flexible needle. A total of 0.2 cc of dexamethasone (8 mg/2 ml) was injected into the left vocal fold. The procedure was well tolerated by the patient with no complications noted. On follow-up 6 weeks later, the patient reported marked improvement in his voice quality. His Voice Handicap Index-10 score dropped from 12 to 3. Laryngeal examination showed partial regression of the edema and the inflammation (Fig. 10.7b). Stroboscopic examination revealed mild improvement in mucosal waves compared to the pre-operative stroboscopic examination.

The patient underwent a second office-based intralesional steroid injection. A total of 0.2 cc of dexamethasone (8 mg/2 ml) was injected into the right vocal fold, and 0.25 cc was injected into the left vocal fold (Fig. 10.7c). The procedure was tolerated well by the patient with no complications noted.

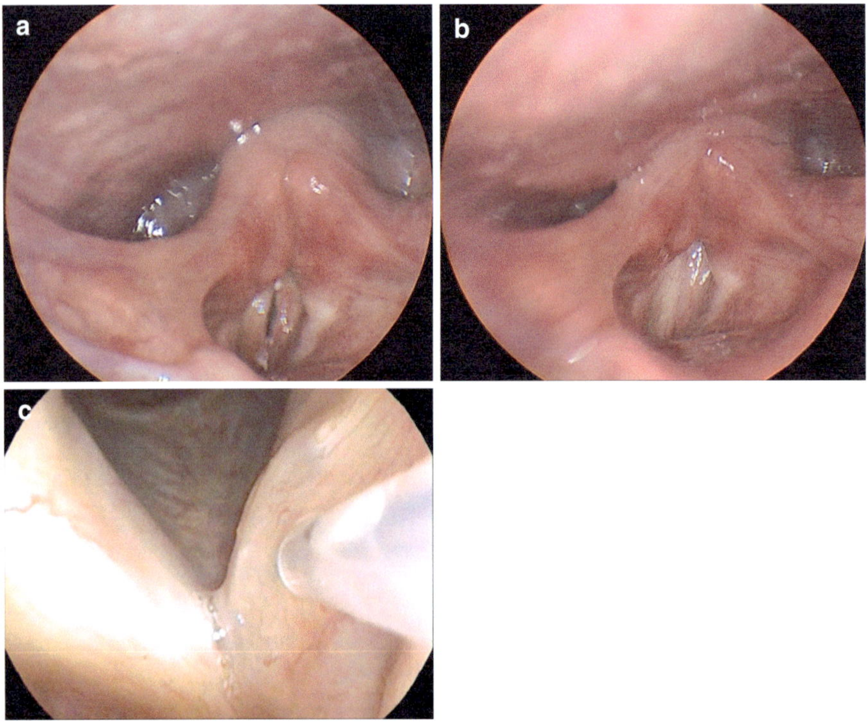

Fig. 10.7 (**a**) An endoscopic view of the larynx showing the leukoplakia on the left vocal fold. Note the edema and inflammation. (**b**) An endoscopic view of the larynx 6 weeks after the vocal fold steroid injection, showing partial decrease in inflammation 6 weeks post-operatively. (**c**) An intra-operative view of the larynx showing the injection of dexamethasone (8 mg/2 ml) into the left vocal fold. Note the submucosal bulge

References

1. Hamdan AL, Sataloff RT, Hawkshaw MJ. Laryngeal manifestations of autoimmune diseases. Laryngeal manifestations of systemic diseases. USA: Plural Publishing; 2019. p. 281.
2. Teitel AD, MacKenzie CR, Stern R, Paget SA. Laryngeal involvement in systemic lupus erythematosus. Semin Arthritis Rheum. 1992;22:203–14.
3. Gilliam JN, Cheatum DE. Immunoglobulins in the larynx in systemic lupus erythematosus. Arch Dermatol. 1973;108(5):696–7.
4. Gómez-Puerta JA, Cisternas A, Hernández MV, Ruiz-Esquide V, Vilaseca I, Sanmartí R. Laryngeal assessment by videolaryngostroboscopy in patients with rheumatoid arthritis. Reumatol Clín (English Ed). 2014;10(1):32–6.
5. Linos A, Worthington JW, O'Fallon MI, Kurland LT. The epidemiology of rheumatoid arthritis in Rochester Minnesota: a study of incidence, prevalence, and mortality. Am J Epidemiol. 1980;111(1):87–98.
6. Lee JH, Sung IY, Park JH, Roh JL. Recurrent laryngeal neuropathy in a systemic lupus erythematosus (SLE) patient. Am J Phys Med Rehabil. 2008;87(1):68–70.

7. Jurik AG, Pedersen U. Rheumatoid arthritis of the crico-arytenoid and crico-thyroid joints: a radiological and clinical study. Clin Radiol. 1984;35(3):233–6.
8. Hosako Y, Nakamura M, Tayama N, Mizuno M, Matunaga A, Niimi S, Hirose H, Hagino S. Laryngeal involvements in systemic lupus erythematosus: a case report. Larynx Jpn. 1993;5:171–5.
9. Perouse R, Coulombeau B, Cornut G, Bouchayer M. "Bamboo nodes": étude clinique à propos de 19 cas ["Bamboo nodes": a clinical study of 19 cases]. Rev Laryngol Otol Rhinol (Bord). 2001;122(5):299–302.
10. Murano E, Hosako-Naito Y, Tayama N, Oka T, Miyaji M, Kumada M, Niimi S. Bamboo node: primary vocal fold lesion as evidence of autoimmune disease. J Voice. 2001;15(3):441–50.
11. Schwemmle C, Ptok M. Bamboo nodes als Ursache von Dysphonien bei Autoimmunkrankheiten [Bamboo nodes as the cause of dysphonias in autoimmune diseases]. HNO. 2007;55(7):564–8. German.
12. Todic J, Schweizer V, Leuchter I. Bamboo nodes of vocal folds: a description of 10 cases and review of the literature. Folia Phoniatr Logop. 2018;70(1):1–7.
13. Lagos AE, García-Huidobro FG, León NI, Napolitano CA, Badía PI. Bamboo nodes as an autoimmune disease laryngeal manifestation. Case series. J Voice. 2023;37(4):636.e1–5.
14. Hamdan AL, Khalifee E, Ghanem A, Mansour H, Yammine E. Predictive value of globus pharyngeus in patients with functional dysphonia versus organic dysphonia. Laryngoscope. 2019;129(4):930–4.
15. Martins RH, do Amaral HA, Tavares EL, Martins MG, Gonçalves TM, Dias NH. Voice disorders: etiology and diagnosis. J Voice. 2016;30(6):761–e1.
16. Sataloff RT, Spiegel JR, Hawkshaw M. Acute mucosal tear and vocal fold hemorrhage. Ear Nose Throat J. 1994;73(9):633.
17. Hoover CA, Sataloff RT, Lyons KM, Hawkshaw M. Vocal fold mucosal tears: maintaining a high clinical index of suspicion. J Voice. 2001;15(3):451–5.

Office-Based Steroid Injection for Vocal Fold Scars and Fibrovascular Masses

11

Vocal fold scar is a common cause of dysphonia that merits special consideration. The etiology is diverse, with the most common cause being injury to the deep structures of the vocal fold following micro-laryngeal surgery. Other causes of vocal fold scar include infectious diseases, inflammatory disorders, neoplastic lesions, and congenital malformations [1]. Blunt or penetrating trauma to the larynx may also result in vocal fold injury and scarring by severing the layered structure of the vocal fold.

Patients with vocal fold scars present with a change in vocal pitch and timbre. Other complaints include voice fatigue and difficulty projecting the voice. The vocal symptoms may be associated with neck pain and throat discomfort secondary to an increase in laryngeal muscle tension. Common findings on flexible laryngoscopy include a trephination or a defect along the upper surface or free edge of the vocal fold and a fibrovascular mass [1]. In patients with penetrating injury to the larynx, vocal fold scar may be associated with a web formation at the anterior commissure, the extent of which varies with the severity of the injury. Stroboscopy invariably shows a decrease or absence of the mucosal waves at the site of the scar. In patients with vocal fold scar and defect, there is incomplete closure of the vocal folds during phonation [2]. *Bouchayer and Cornut* classified vocal fold scars based on severity of the disease into various categories ranging from notching of the vocal fold to fibrous scarring with rigidity [3].

The phonatory symptoms and stroboscopic findings in patients with vocal fold scars are attributed to injury to the deep structures of the vocal fold, namely remodeling of the extracellular matrix (ECM) constituents of the lamina propria and alterations in the viscoelastic properties of the fold [4]. In 2002, Thibault et al. investigated the histologic and rheologic properties of the scarred vocal fold in a

Supplementary Information The online version contains supplementary material available at https://doi.org/10.1007/978-3-032-05235-3_11.

A. L. Hamdan, *Atlas of Office-based Laryngeal Steroid Injection*,
https://doi.org/10.1007/978-3-032-05235-3_11

rabbit model. The authors reported an increase in procollagen and a decrease in elastin 60 days following injury. The authors also noted increase in stiffness ascribed to disorganized collagen bundles in the lamina propria [5]. In 2005, Rousseau et al. examined the long-term histological properties of the scarred vocal fold in a canine model and reported a decrease in elastin fibers and an increase in procollagen 2 months following injury. The decrease in elastin—which became tangled—was persistent at 6 months and was accompanied by an increase in thick and disorganized collagen fibers [6]. In 2014, Hu et al. investigated the expression of ECM proteins in injured vocal folds in a canine model using immunofluorescence staining. The authors reported an increase in fibronectin at 2 months following injury. Fibronectin is a glycoprotein present primarily in the intermediate and deep layer of the lamina propria and helps in binding the other proteins to strengthen the ECM [7].

Treatment of vocal fold scarring is a challenging task. Voice therapy (VT) and control of confounding risk factors, such as reflux disease, are often a good start. The purpose of voice therapy is to restore the malleability of vocal fold cover and to reduce the compensatory hyper-functional laryngeal behavior that is often present in affected patients. The success rate of VT is usually low, particularly in patients with a long-standing history of vocal fold scarring. In patients who fail voice therapy, surgery is often recommended.

Several surgical techniques have been described in the literature. These include excision of the fibrous tissue or scar, serial mucosal slicing, severance of adhesions between the mucosal cover and underlying lamina propria, insertion of a scaffold using decellularized matrix, biological or synthetic polymers, use of fascial implants, collagen injection, fat injection, and application of topical mitomycin [8–13]. Injection laryngoplasty and thyroplasty are also commonly performed to improve glottic closure in patients with vocal fold scar and glottic insufficiency. It is important to note that laryngeal framework surgery does not address the histologic changes and viscoelastic properties of the scarred vocal fold [14, 15].

With the shift in laryngology practice from the operating room to the clinic, many cases of vocal fold scar are treated in-office under local anesthesia. Several treatment options are offered to the patient. These include laser therapy and injection of pharmaceutical agents such as glucocorticoids, and hyaluronic acid [16–18]. Laser therapy stimulates the activity of the fibroblasts, which are primarily responsible for maintaining the structural support of the lamina propria and its functional properties [18, 19]. Steroid therapy modulates the inflammatory response following injury, inhibits cellular proliferation; thus reducing the synthesis of collagen [20]. Their anti-inflammatory effect is mediated via regulation of cytokine production and other inflammatory mediators, both at the cellular and genetic levels [21].

In 2002, Carroll et al. conducted a study on human dermal fibroblasts and noted that injection of 20 μm of triamcinolone acetonide increased the production of basic fibroblast growth factor and decreased the production of transforming growth factor beta 1 (TGF-beta1) [22].

In 2006, Mortensen and Woo reported significant improvement in the overall grade of dysphonia following Intralesional Steroid Injections (ILSI) in 12 patients with vocal fold scar. The improvement in voice quality following the injection was associated with an increase in mucosal waves and amplitude on stroboscopy. The authors concluded that office-based steroid injection is an efficacious treatment option in patients with vocal fold scar, and other benign lesions of the vocal folds [23].

In 2011, Woo et al. analyzed the efficacy of percutaneous steroid injection in the treatment of benign lesions of the vocal folds in a cohort of 115 patients and noted a subjective and objective improvement in 84.4% of their study group, which included 13 cases of vocal fold scar [24].

In 2016, Young et al. reviewed their case series of 25 patients with mild/moderate vocal fold scars who underwent office-based dexamethasone injection, and reported improvement in subjective and objective voice outcome measures 13.7 ± 4.4 weeks following treatment. There was a significant decrease in the Voice Handicap Index (VHI) score, and the GRBAS ratings associated with a significant improvement in glottic closure and mucosal waves on stroboscopy [25].

In 2023, Kruse et al. evaluated the effect of three-times office-based steroid injections in a cohort of 23 patients with vocal fold scars who also pursued voice therapy. There was a significant decrease in the Voice Handicap Index (VHI) score, and auditory perceptual rating. The subjective improvement was accompanied by an increase in the mucosal waves and normalization of the free edge of the vocal folds. Although the Phonatory Threshold Pressure (PTP) and glottic closure did not improve, the authors advocated ILSI, particularly in patients who refuse surgical intervention [26].

With the advances in basic science and our better understanding of the dynamic behavior of the lamina propria, new treatment alternatives for vocal fold scars, aside from ILSI and laser therapy, are gaining ground. One of these is tissue engineering. This latter has emerged as a new approach to treat severe vocal fold scar by modulating the activity of cells within the lamina propria via regulatory factors. Tissue engineering relies on the stimulation of ECM cells to restore the pre-morbid architectural landscape of the lamina propria. Examples include the use of growth factors to improve fibroblast activity. Fibroblast growth factors have been shown to stimulate hyaluronic acid (HA) production and reduce collagen type 1 formation [27, 28].

Cell therapy is another form of tissue regenerative therapy that helps restore the lamina propria constituents. An example is the implantation of stem cells within scarred vocal folds with the aim of improving wound healing, and the vibratory characteristics of the vocal fold [29].

11.1 Case 1

A 48-year-old man, a heavy smoker, presented to the Voice Clinic with a history of voice fatigue and loss of the high notes, the patient reported a history of voice overuse. His Voice Handicap Index-10 (VHI-10) score was 10. Acoustic analysis revealed, a habitual pitch (HP) of 131.84 Hz, jitter of 0.88, shimmer of 3.1, a noise-to-harmonics ratio (NHR) of 0.10, and a voice turbulence index (VTI) of 0.043. His maximum phonation time (MPT) was 17.3 s. Laryngeal endoscopic examination revealed bilateral vocal fold scarring. On stroboscopic examination, there was a decrease in mucosal waves bilaterally with incomplete closure of the vocal folds during phonation (Fig. 11.1a; Video 11.1a).

The patient underwent office-based steroid injection. A 0.1 cc of dexamethasone (8 mg/2 ml) was injected into the right vocal fold, and 0.2 cc into the left vocal fold. The procedure was performed using a 25-gauge flexible needle that was inserted into the working channel of the flexible endoscope (Fig. 11.1b). The procedure was tolerated well by the patient with no complications noted.

On follow-up 3 weeks later, the patient improved his voice quality. His VHI-10 score dropped to 2. Acoustic analysis revealed a habitual pitch (HP) of 137.94 Hz, jitter of 0.906, shimmer of 2.061, a noise-to-harmonics ratio (NHR) of 0.094 and a voice turbulence index (VTI) of 0.044. His maximum phonation time (MPT) was 22.51 s. Laryngeal examination revealed partial regression of the vocal fold scarring (Fig. 11.1c; Video 11.1b).

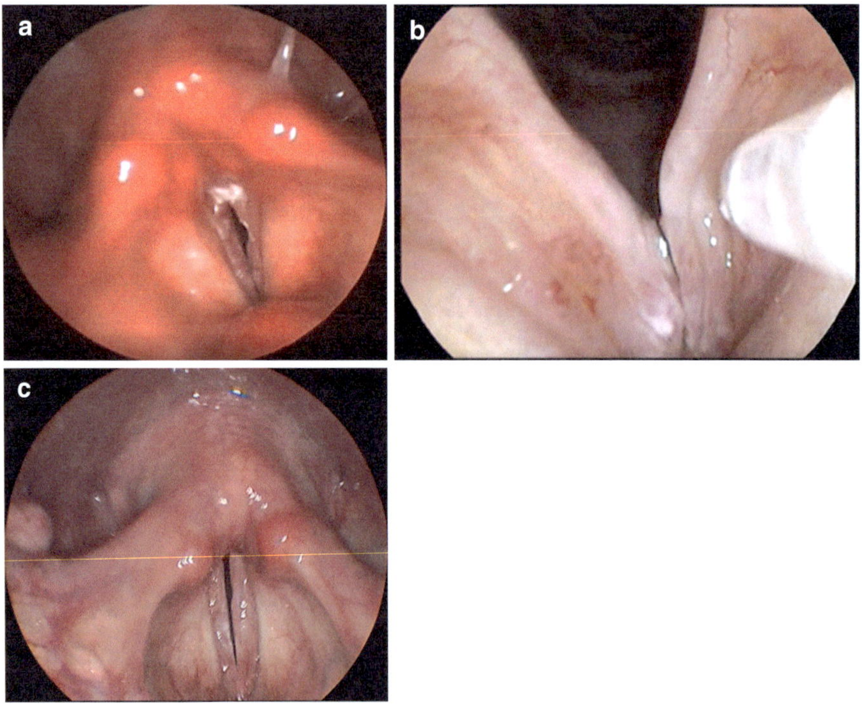

Fig. 11.1 (**a**) Preoperative endoscopic view of the larynx showing bilateral vocal fold scarring with incomplete closure of the vocal folds. (**b**) An endoscopic view of the larynx showing the insertion of the needle in the left vocal fold scar tissue. Note the bleb formation. (**c**) A stroboscopic view of the larynx showing a decrease in vocal fold scarring

11.2 Case 2

A 59-year-old woman presented to the voice clinic with persistent dysphonia following microlaryngeal surgery for bilateral Reinke's edema. The patient was a former smoker and had no history of allergy or reflux disease. She had a history of a previous office-based laser therapy and vocal fold steroid injection 1 year before her presentation. Her Voice Handicap Index-10 (VHI-10) score was 25. Acoustic analysis revealed a fundamental frequency (F0) of 262.51 Hz, jitter of 3.6, shimmer of 16.8, a noise-to-harmonics ratio (NHR) of 0.313, and a voice turbulence index (VTI) of 0.063. Her maximum phonation time (MPT) was 7.7 s. Laryngeal endoscopic examination revealed bilateral vocal fold scarring (Fig. 11.2a).

The patient underwent serial office-based steroid injections (dexamethasone [8 mg/2 ml] over 9 months. The injections were made using the transnasal approach (Fig. 11.2b, c; Video 11.2).

On her last follow-up, the patient reported marked improvement in voice quality. Her VHI-10 score dropped to 3. Acoustic analysis revealed a fundamental frequency (F0) of 207.021 Hz, jitter of 1.27, shimmer of 5.73, a noise-to-harmonics ratio (NHR) of 0.129, and a voice turbulence index (VTI) of 0.053. Her maximum phonation time (MPT) was 10.04 s. Laryngeal examination showed marked decrease in vocal fold scarring.

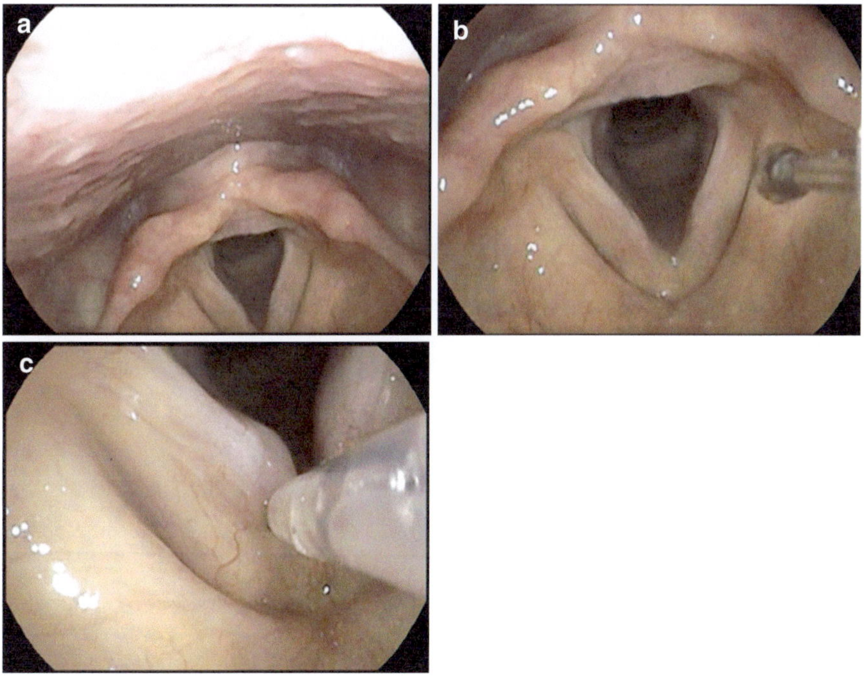

Fig. 11.2 (**a**) An endoscopic view of the larynx showing bilateral vocal fold scarring. (**b**) An endoscopic view showing the tip of the needle directed toward the left vocal fold. (**c**) An intraoperative view showing the needle inserted into the right vocal fold Reinke's space. Note the bleb formation

11.3 Case 3

A 44-year-old man, a heavy smoker, presented to the voice clinic with a history of dysphonia of a few months' duration. His medical history was negative for reflux disease or allergy. His Voice Handicap Index-10 (VHI-10) score at presentation was 28. Acoustic analysis revealed a fundamental frequency (F0) of 116.03 Hz, habitual pitch (HP) of 118.29 Hz, jitter of 0.652, shimmer of 2.61, a noise-to-harmonics ratio (NHR) of 0.135, and a voice turbulence index (VTI) of 0.049. His maximum phonation time (MPT) was 29.07 s. Laryngeal endoscopic examination revealed chronic inflammatory changes and fibrosis with a whitish lesion on the upper surface of the left vocal fold near the anterior commissure (Fig. 11.3a).

The patient underwent multiple office-based steroid injections between December 2019 and May 2024. The dose injected ranged from 0.15 cc to 0.6 cc of dexamethasone (8 mg/2 ml) using a 25-gauge flexible needle that was introduced through the working channel of a flexible endoscope (Fig. 11.3b–d; Video 11.3). All procedures were tolerated well by the patient with no complications noted.

The patient reported mild improvement in voice quality after each injection. His Voice Handicap Index-10 (VHI-10) score decreased to 10. Acoustic analysis revealed an increase in his fundamental frequency (F0) of 126.53 Hz, habitual pitch (HP) of 122.55 Hz, a decrease in jitter of 0.48, shimmer of 2.049, noise-to-harmonics ratio (NHR) 0.12, and voice turbulence index (VTI) of 0.039. His maximum phonation time (MPT) increased to 26.27 s. Laryngeal examination following the last ILSI showed marked improvement in the vocal fold cover malleability and closure during phonation (Fig. 11.3e, f).

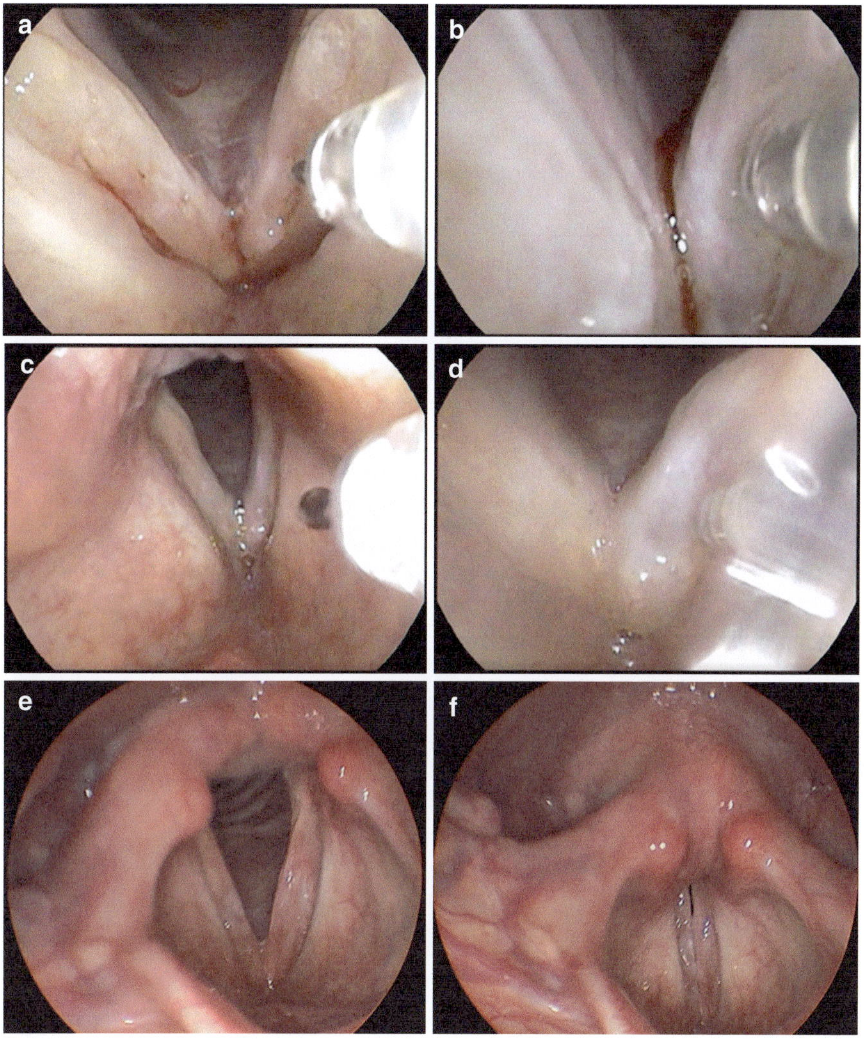

Fig. 11.3 (**a**) Endoscopic view of the larynx showing scarring of both vocal folds. Note the small polypoidal mass on the upper surface of the left vocal fold near the anterior commissure. (**b**) An endoscopic view of the larynx showing left vocal fold ILSI. (**c**) An endoscopic view of the larynx following the third intralesional steroid injection. (**d**) An endoscopic view showing a bleb formation following the ILSI. (**e**) A stroboscopic view of the larynx following ILSI showing marked reduction in fibrosis. (**f**) A stroboscopic view of the larynx showing complete closure of the vocal folds during phonation. Note persistent edema and scarring of both vocal folds

11.4 Case 4

A 69-year-old man presented to the voice clinic with voice fatigue and a decrease in vocal range. He had a positive history of reflux disease that was treated empirically. He denied any history of smoking or allergy. Laryngeal examination revealed bilateral vocal fold scarring with right vocal fold hemorrhage.

The patient was advised voice rest and was prescribed a course of steroids (predictor 40 mg once daily for 4 days, followed by 20 mg for 4 days). Endoscopic examination 9 months later showed scarring of the vocal folds with a decrease in mucosal waves on stroboscopy. The hemorrhage had resolved.

The patient was advised to undergo an office-based intralesional steroid injection (Fig. 11.4a). His Voice Handicap Index-10 (VHI-10) score before the injection was 7. The injection was performed using the transnasal approach. A 25-gauge needle was introduced into the working channel of the scope, and a total of 0.2 cc of dexamethasone (8 mg/2 ml) was injected into the left vocal fold, and 0.3 cc was injected into the right vocal fold (Fig. 11.4b–d). The procedure was tolerated well by the patient with no complications.

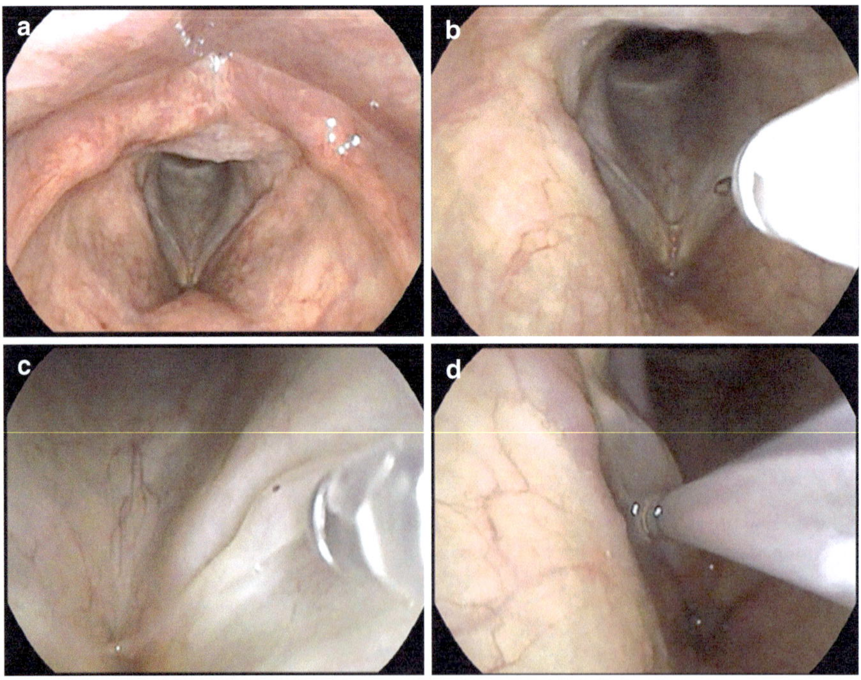

Fig. 11.4 (**a**) An endoscopic view of the larynx prior to the steroid injection showing bilateral vocal fold scarring. (**b**) An endoscopic view while directing the needle toward the left vocal fold. (**c**) An endoscopic view showing left vocal fold intralesional steroid injection. (**d**) An endoscopic view of the larynx showing a bleb in the right vocal fold following steroid injection

11.5 Case 5

A 79-year-old woman, a smoker, presented to the voice clinic with persistent hoarseness following microlaryngeal surgery performed in an outside hospital. The patient denied any history of phonotrauma, allergy, or reflux disease. Her Voice Handicap Index-10 (VHI-10) score at presentation was 21. Acoustic analysis revealed a fundamental frequency (F0) of 174.8 Hz, habitual pitch (HP) of 246.18 Hz, jitter of 4.54, shimmer of 8.6, a noise-to-harmonics ratio (NHR) of 0.315, and a voice turbulence index (VTI) of 0.112. Her maximum phonation time (MPT) was 6.34 s. Laryngeal flexible endoscopic examination revealed right vocal fold scarring with severe inflammation and residual polypoid tissue on the left vocal fold (Fig. 11.5a).

The patient underwent office-based steroid injection into both vocal folds using the transnasal approach (Fig. 11.5b, c). The procedure was well tolerated by the patient with no complications noted. On follow-up 4 weeks later, the patient had marked improvement in her voice quality. Her VHI-10 score dropped to 3. Acoustic

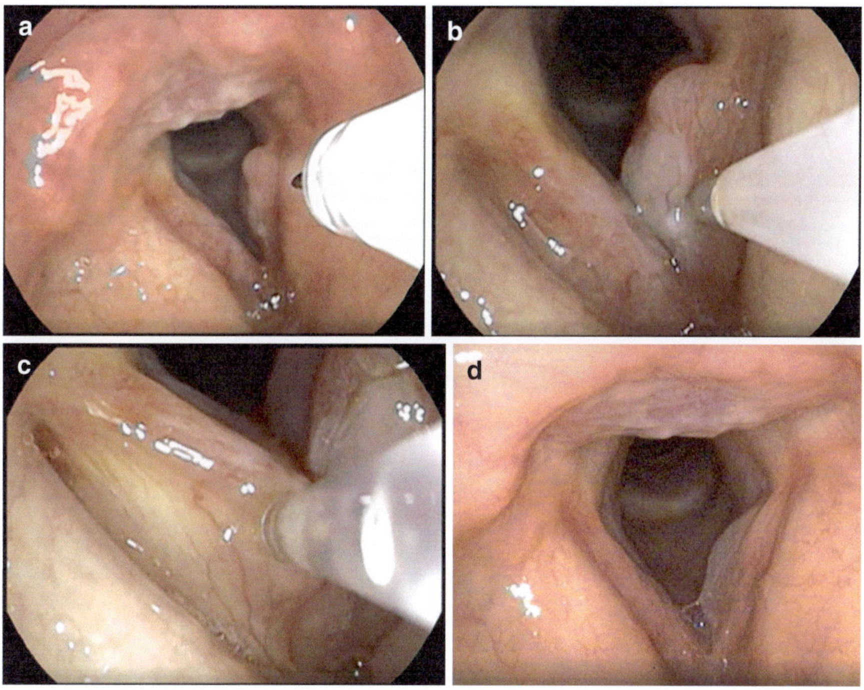

Fig. 11.5 (**a**) Intraoperative view of the larynx before the injection showing inflammation and fibrosis of both vocal folds. (**b**) An endoscopic view of the larynx showing left vocal fold steroid injection using the transnasal approach. (**c**) An endoscopic view of the larynx showing right vocal fold steroid injection using the transnasal approach. (**d**) Endoscopic view of the larynx 4 weeks following ILSI for both vocal folds showing a decrease in redness and edema of both vocal folds. Note the persistence of residual disease on the left vocal folds

analysis showed a decrease in F0 to 135.74 Hz, HP to 109.65 Hz, and jitter of 1.7 (Fig. 11.5d). The patient was advised to undergo repeated vocal fold steroid injections and voice therapy.

11.6 Case 6

A 71-year-old man presented to the voice clinic with hoarseness of a few months' duration. The patient has a positive history of tonsillar tumor and underwent radiation therapy 8 years ago. He has a positive history of smoking and phonotrauma. He denied any history of reflux disease or allergy. His Voice Handicap Index-10 (VHI-10) score on presentation was 27. Flexible laryngoscopy scarring of both vocal folds (due to radiation) in addition to leukoplakia on the free edge of both vocal folds anteriorly (Fig. 11.6a). The patient had also medialization of the false vocal folds during phonation (muscle tension pattern type II), suggestive of secondary muscle tension dysphonia (Fig. 11.6b).

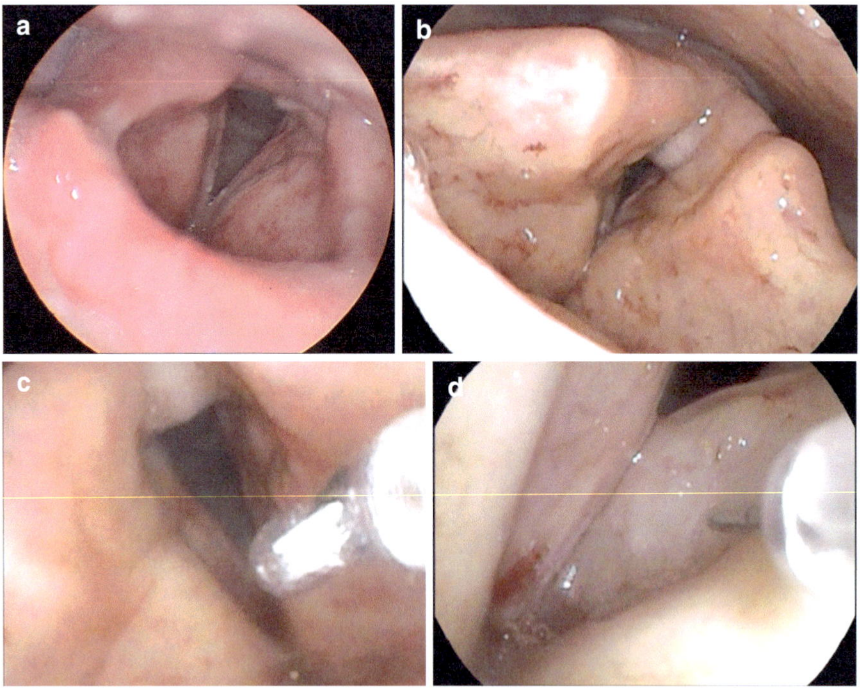

Fig. 11.6 (**a**) An endoscopic view of the larynx showing bilateral lesions of the vocal folds. (**b**) An endoscopic view of the larynx showing a muscle tension pattern type II. (**c**) An endoscopic view of the larynx showing the cup forceps directed towards the right vocal fold. (**d**) An endoscopic intraoperative view showing the injection of dexamethasone (8 mg/2 ml). Note the fullness and blanching at the site of injection

The patient underwent office-based biopsy of the vocal fold lesions. Histopathologic examination showed mild acute inflammation with no dysplasia (Fig. 11.6c).

The patient was advised voice therapy and bilateral vocal folds steroid injections. The procedure was performed via the transnasal approach using the 25-gauge flexible needle. A total of 0.2 cc of dexamethasone (8 mg/2 ml) was injected into each vocal fold (Fig. 11.6d). The procedure was tolerated well by the patient with no complications noted.

References

1. Benninger MS, Alessi D, Archer S, Bastian R, Ford C, Koufman J, Sataloff RT, Spiegel JR, Woo P. Vocal fold scarring: current concepts and management. Otolaryngol Head Neck Surg. 1996;115(5):474–82.
2. Hantzakos A, Dikkers FG, Giovanni A, Benninger MS, Remacle M, Sjögren EV, Woo P. Vocal fold scars: a common classification proposal by the American Laryngological Association and European Laryngological Society. Eur Arch Otorrinolaringol. 2019;276:2289–92.
3. Bouchayer M, Cornut G. Microsurgical treatment of benign vocal fold lesions: indications, technique, results. Folia Phoniatr Logop. 1992;44(3–4):155–84.
4. Leydon C, Imaizumi M, Bartlett RS, et al. Epithelial cells are active participants in vocal fold wound healing: an in vivo animal model of injury. PLoS One. 2014;9(12):e115389.
5. Thibeault SL, Gray SD, Bless DM, Chan RW, Ford CN. Histologic and rheologic characterization of vocal fold scarring. J Voice. 2002;16(1):96–104.
6. Rousseau B, Hirano S, Scheidt TD, Welham NV, Thibeault SL, Chan RW, Bless DM. Characterization of vocal fold scarring in a canine model. Laryngoscope. 2003;113(4):620–7.
7. Hu R, Xu W, Ling W, Wang Q, Wu Y, Han D. Characterization of extracellular matrix proteins during wound healing in the lamina propria of vocal fold in a canine model: a long-term and consecutive study. Acta Histochem. 2014;116(5):730–5.
8. Tsunoda K, Baer T, Niimi S. Autologous transplantation of fascia into the vocal fold: long term results of a new phonosurgical technique for glottal incompetence. Laryngoscope. 2001;111:453–7.
9. Kishimoto Y, Hirano S, Kojima T, Kanemaru SI, Ito J. Implantation of an atelocollagen sheet for the treatment of vocal fold scarring and sulcus vocalis. Ann Otol Rhinol Laryngol. 2009;118:613–20.
10. Karle WE, Helman SN, Cooper A, Zhang Y, Pitman MJ. Temporalis fascia transplantation for sulcus vocalis and vocal fold scar: long-term outcomes. Ann Otol Rhinol Laryngol. 2018;127:223–8.
11. Kairys SW, Olmstead EM, O'Connor GT. Steroid treatment oflaryngotracheitis: a meta-analysis of the evidence fromrandomized trials. Pediatrics. 1989;83:683–93.
12. Ossoff RH, Wolff AP, Ballenger JJ. Acute epiglottitis inadults: experience with fifteen cases. Laryngoscope. 1980;90:1155–61.
13. Ridder GJ, Strohhacker H, Lohle E, et al. Laryngeal sarcoid-osis: treatment with the antileprosy drug clofazimine. Ann Otol Rhinol Laryngol. 2000;109:1146–9.
14. Ford CN, Staskowski PA, Bless DM. Autologous collagen vocal fold injection: a preliminary clinical study. Laryngoscope. 1995;105:944–8.
15. Remacle M, Lawson G, Hedayat A, et al. Medialization framework surgery for voice improvement after endoscopic cordectomy. Eur Arch Otorrinolaringol. 2001;258:267–71.
16. Chan RW, Gray SD, Titze IR. The importance of hyaluronic acid in vocal fold biomechanics. Otolaryngol Head Neck Surg. 2001;124:607–14.

17. Dahlqvist A, Garskog O, Laurent C, et al. Viscoelasticity of rabbit vocal folds after injection augmentation. Laryngoscope. 2004;114:138–42. This paper revealed good viscoelasticity of hyaluronan-implanted vocal folds.
18. Bouchayer M, Cornut G. Microsurgery for benign lesions of the vocal folds. Ear Nose Throat J. 1988;67:446–66.
19. Woo P, Casper J, Colton R, et al. Diagnosis and treatment of persistent dysphonia after laryngeal surgery: a retrospective analysis of 62 patients. Laryngoscope. 1994;104:1084–91.
20. Wang CT, Liao LJ, Cheng PW, Lo WC, Lai MS. Intralesional steroid injection for benign vocal fold disorders: a systematic review and meta-analysis. Laryngoscope. 2013;123(1):197–203.
21. Hardison S. Medical management. In: Moore JE, Sataloff RT, Hawkshaw M, editors. Vocal Fold Scar: current concepts and management. London: Compton Publishing; 2016. p. 54–62.
22. Carroll LA, Hanasono MM, Mikulec AA, Kita M, Koch RJ. Triamcinolone stimulates bFGF production and inhibits TGF-β1 production by human dermal fibroblasts. Dermatologic Surg. 2002;28(8):704–9.
23. Mortensen M, Woo P. Office steroid injections of the larynx. Laryngoscope. 2006;116(10):1735–9.
24. Woo JH, Kim DY, Kim JW, Oh EA, Lee SW. Efficacy of percutaneous vocal fold injections for benign laryngeal lesions: prospective multicenter study. Acta Otolaryngol. 2011;131(12):1326–32.
25. Young WG, Hoffman MR, Koszewski IJ, Whited CW, Ruel BN, Dailey SH. Voice outcomes following a single office-based steroid injection for vocal fold scar. Otolaryngol Head Neck Surg. 2016;155(5):820–8.
26. Kruse CM, Hoffman MR, Hennessy BN, Schoeff SS, Dailey SH. Voice outcomes following serial office-based steroid injections and voice therapy for vocal fold scar. J Voice. 2023:S0892-1997(23)00093-0. https://doi.org/10.1016/j.jvoice.2023.02.036. Epub ahead of print. PMID: 37076383.
27. Hirano S, Bless D, Heisey D, et al. Roles of hepatocyte growth factor and transforming growth factor beta1 in production of extracellular matrix by canine vocal fold fibroblasts. Laryngoscope. 2003;113:144–8.
28. Hirano S, Bless DM, Rousseau B, et al. Prevention of vocal fold scarring by topical injection of hepatocyte growth factor in rabbit model. Laryngoscope. 2004;114:548–56.
29. Kanemaru S, Nakamura T, Omori K, et al. Regeneration of the vocal fold using autologous mesenchymal stem cells. Ann Otol Rhinol Laryngol. 2003;112:915–20.

Office-Based Steroid Injection in Subglottic Stenosis

12

Subglottic stenosis (SGS) is a form of partial or complete narrowing of the laryngeal airway [1]. The stenotic segment is in the subglottic region but may extend caudally to the trachea, resulting in laryngotracheal stenosis. The stenosis may also extend cephalically to the glottis, leading to narrowing of the glottic aperture with or without impairment in the mobility of the vocal folds. Subglottic stenosis accounts for 50% of laryngotracheal stenosis, the prevalence of which is 1 in 200,000 adults [2, 3]. Affected patients invariably present with respiratory complaints that are falsely ascribed to diseases of the lower airway. The most commonly reported symptoms are dyspnea, wheezing, cough, and stridor. In severe cases, patients may present with respiratory distress—necessitating a tracheotomy to secure the airway.

The etiology of subglottic stenosis is complex and multifactorial. The most common cause is iatrogenic injury, accounting for 50% of the cases [1, 4]. The trauma can occur during the insertion of an endotracheal tube or following a prolonged intubation. High contact pressure from the cuff and/or the distal tip of the tube leads to vascular compression of the surrounding tissues with subsequent ulceration and scar formation (Fig. 12.1).

Numerous studies indicate that the use of an endotracheal tube greater than 7.5 mm is one of many risk factors implicated in the pathogenesis of SGS [5, 6]. Following injury to the mucosal lining, three stages of wound healing develop, leading to fibrosis and scar formation. These include inflammation, proliferation, and maturation [7–13]. Other rare causes of SGS include external trauma to the neck, infectious and autoimmune diseases such as granulomatosis with polyangiitis (Fig. 12.2) [7].

Supplementary Information The online version contains supplementary material available at https://doi.org/10.1007/978-3-032-05235-3_12.

A. L. Hamdan, *Atlas of Office-based Laryngeal Steroid Injection*,
https://doi.org/10.1007/978-3-032-05235-3_12

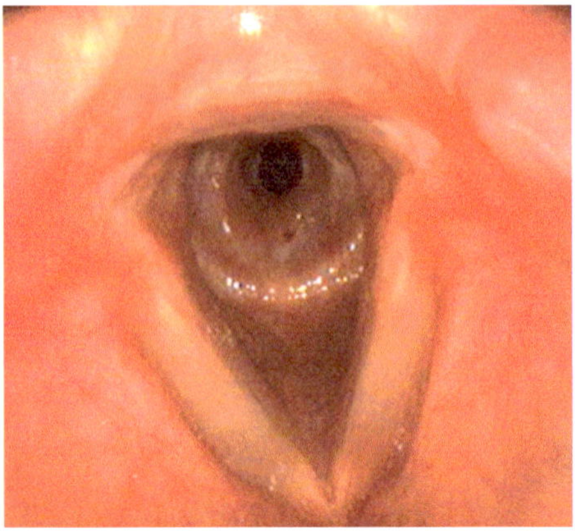

Fig. 12.1 An endoscopic view showing laryngotracheal stenosis

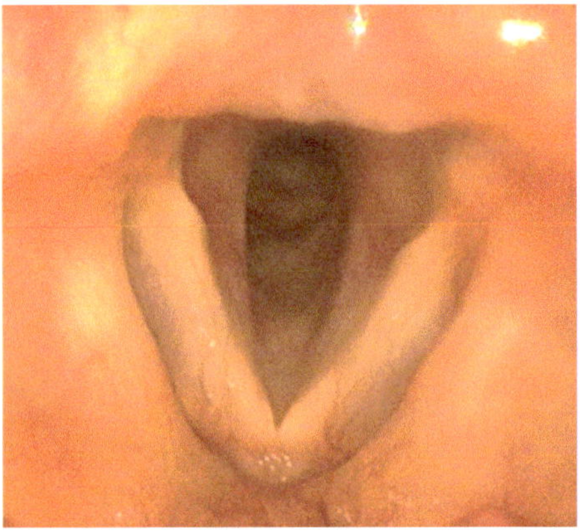

Fig. 12.2 Case of polyangiitis granulomatosis presenting with shortness of breath, of years duration. On laryngeal examination, she has subglottic stenosis

In the absence of any clear inciting cause, SGS is labeled as idiopathic. Idiopathic subglottic stenosis (ISGS) is a progressive form of laryngeal inflammatory disorder that occurs exclusively in women. The pathophysiology of this devastating condition remains unclear, and the true etiology is still not fully understood. One suggested hypothesis is dysregulation in the immune response [14].

The diagnosis of SGS is not always easy. Based on numerous studies, the average delay in diagnosis can extend up to 4 years, as most patients are commonly treated for asthma or other respiratory diseases [15–17]. Pulmonary function testing, particularly the expiratory disproportion index (EDI) (defined as the ratio of forced expiratory flow in 1 s to peak expiratory flow rate), is commonly used to differentiate between SGS and diseases of the lower airway. Nouraei et al. reported a moderate correlation between the severity of SGS and EDI, which had a sensitivity and specificity of 95.9% and 94.2%, respectively [18]. Imaging studies using computed tomography or magnetic resonance can also help delineate the lumen of the subglottic region and the vertical height of the stenotic segment [19]. Dynamic expiratory computed tomography is also useful in gauging the dynamic behavior of the larynx and trachea [20]. Endoscopic visualization of the subglottic region in an awake setting or under light anesthesia remains the best method to assess the severity of stenosis, as well as any collapse in the airway.

Treatment of SGS is very challenging, given the complexity of this condition. A multidisciplinary approach is often needed to address the respiratory, phonatory and swallowing symptoms in affected patients. A speech-language pathologist, a pulmonologist, and an otolaryngologist are frequently engaged in treatment. Various surgical procedures are offered to the patient, taking into account the stage of the disease and its severity. These options include laryngotracheoplasty which consists of airway augmentation using various types of grafts or expanders, with or without dilation; laryngotracheal resection, which involves end-to-end anastomosis; and tracheotomy [1].

Given the considerable rate of recurrence, which varies between 40% and 70% [21], monotherapy with surgery has been questioned, and new therapeutic modalities have been introduced, including steroid injections. The use of intralesional steroids has expanded following its successful application in the treatment of scars and keloids in dermatology. The decrease in fibrosis and scar formation is due to their anti-inflammatory effect. There is a decrease in the level of inflammatory markers—such as cytokines and interleukin-10—and a decrease in the migration of inflammatory cells. Glucocorticoids also have an antimitotic activity, which results in a decrease in fibroblast proliferation, leading to a decrease in the synthesis of collagen and other glycosaminoglycans [22–24]. Another suggested mechanism is vasoconstriction, which reduces the blood supply to the scar tissue, leading to hypoxia and scar regression.

There is expanding literature on the use of serial steroid injections as a primary or adjuvant treatment of SGS following surgery. With the reform in laryngology practice—from the operating room to the clinic—intralesional steroid injections (ILSI) are commonly performed under local anesthesia, with promising results.

In 2017, Hoffman et al. reviewed their experience in 19 patients with idiopathic subglottic stenosis who were treated with serial steroid injections in an office setting. The completion rate was 98.8% and no complications were noted. Injection of steroids at least three times obviated the need for surgical intervention in the operating room in 14 out of 17 patients. In those who underwent two sets of three injections, the average stenosis decreased from 40% ± 15% pre-operatively to 25% ± 10% post-operatively [25].

In 2017, Franco Jr. et al. conducted a retrospective study comparing office-based serial ILSI to endoscopic treatment in the operating room, followed by office-based ILSI in a cohort of 13 patients with ISGS. Both groups had significant improvement in breathing associated with an increase in % peak expiratory flow (PEF). Eighty percent of the group treated in-office alone had sustained % PEF above 80% in comparison to 86% in those treated in the operating room and office. The difference between the two groups was not statistically significant [14].

In 2018, Wolianky et al. investigated the systemic effect of steroid injections in six patients with ISGS who had a single injection of triamcinolone ranging between 40 and 200 mg. The authors noted a decline in both systemic and salivary cortisol level at day 1 following the injection, which normalized after a week, with no cumulative effect seen at day 28. The authors attributed this decline to an acute suppression of the hypothalamic-pituitary-adrenal axis. The inflammatory markers did not exhibit any significant changes [26].

In 2019, Pan and Rosow et al. investigated the impact of adjuvant ILSI on surgery-free-intervals (SFI) in 13 patients who underwent endoscopic dilation and at least one steroid injection in an office setting. The surgery-free interval increased from 288.6 ± 362 days to 545.5 ± 152.7 days (p value 0.0041). The average number of injections was 4.2, and the mean follow-up period was 20.4 months. The authors concluded that ILSI is a valuable adjuvant treatment modality to surgery and helps expand SFIs [27].

In 2020, Hoffman et al. investigated the severity of dyspnea in 16 patients with mild-to-moderate stenosis who underwent three ILSIs and found a significant decrease in the dyspnea index score and in the Modified Medical Research Council (MMRC) dyspnea scale score as well. The main side effects were temporary airway restriction and cough noted in five and three cases, respectively. There was no significant change in the Voice Handicap Index-10 (VHI-1O) score following treatment [28].

In 2023, Luke et al. conducted a systematic review of the literature on the efficacy of ILSI in the management of subglottic stenosis and noted an increase in SFI from 362.9 to 582.2 days following treatment. Only one-fourth of the participants in their review (41 out of 55) required further surgical intervention. The authors reaffirmed the safety of this treatment modality and its efficacy in reducing the rate of surgical intervention [29].

In 2023, Schoeff et al. examined the long-term effect of ILSI in 57 patients and noted that those who had an injection following endoscopic dilation had a longer interoperative interval than those who underwent dilation alone. The increase in interoperative interval was associated with a decrease in the extent of stenosis and dyspnea [30].

In 2024, Schuering et al. investigated the added value of ILSI in patients undergoing endoscopic dilation compared to a subgroup who had been previously treated with endoscopic dilation alone. The results showed an increase of 6 months in the time until reintervention. The authors concluded that ILSI is an effective adjuvant treatment to endoscopic dilation that helps prolong the interval before surgical intervention in patients with autoimmune or idiopathic subglottic stenosis [31].

12.1 Case 1

A 26-year-old woman presented to the voice clinic with hoarseness and shortness of breath following a prolonged intubation. Her Voice Handicap Index 10 (VHI-10) score was 19. Her Dyspnea Severity Index (DSI) was 20. Acoustic analysis revealed a fundamental frequency (F0) of 212.25 Hz, habitual pitch (HP) of 188.25 Hz, jitter of 2, shimmer of 3.76, a noise-to-harmonics ratio (NHR) of 0.147, and a Voice Turbulence Index (VTI) of 0.079. Her maximum phonation time (MPT) was 7.86.

Laryngeal flexible examination revealed a subglottic edema and scarring extending to the trachea. Computed tomography (CT) scan of the neck showed mild cricoid cartilage erosion on the left side with formation of granulation tissue, causing 50% narrowing of the subglottic airway.

The patient underwent an office-based steroid injection under local anesthesia. A total of 0.15 cc of dexamethasone (8 mg/2 ml) was injected into the subglottic/tracheal scar (Fig. 12.3a, b; Video 12.1a). The procedure was tolerated well by the patient with no complications noted.

On follow-up 4 weeks later, the patient had marked improvement in her breathing and voice quality. Her VHI-10 score dropped to 1, and her DSI score dropped to 0. Acoustic analysis showed an increase in the F0 to 216.98 Hz. There was a decrease in jitter of 1.12 and in shimmer to 2. There was an increase in her MPT to 10.8 s. Laryngeal examination revealed marked improvement with mild residual disease.

The patient underwent a second office-based steroid injection. A total of 0.2 cc of dexamethasone (8 mg/2 ml) was injected into the tracheal scar (Fig. 12.3c; Video 12.1b).

The procedure was tolerated well by the patient with no complications noted. Follow-up 6 weeks later showed marked disease regression and widening of the airway (Fig. 12.3d).

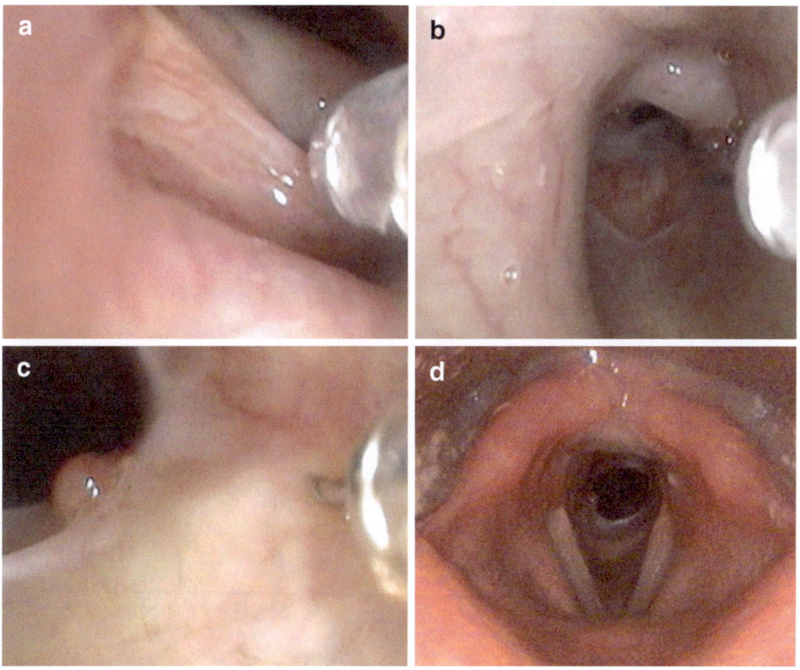

Fig. 12.3 (**a**) An endoscopic view showing the injection of 0.1–0.2 ml of dexamethasone into the scar tissue. (**b**) An endoscopic view of the larynx showing the needle directed toward the tracheal stenotic segment. (**c**) Endoscopic view showing injection of steroid into the scar tissue. Note the blanching of the mucosa after the injection. (**d**) Endoscopic view 1 month after the second injection showing marked disease regression

References

1. Pasick LJ, Anis MM, Rosow DE. An updated review of subglottic stenosis: etiology, evaluation, and management. Curr Pulmonol Rep. 2022;11(2):29–38.
2. Nouraei SAR, Ma E, Patel A, Howard DJ, Sandhu GS. Estimating the population incidence of adult post-intubation laryngotracheal stenosis. Clin Otolaryngol. 2007;32:411–2.
3. Poetker DM, Ettema SL, Blumin JH, Toohill RJ, Merati AL. Association of airway abnormalities and risk factors in 37 subglottic stenosis patients. Otolaryngol Head Neck Surg. 2006;135:434–7.
4. Gelbard A, Francis DO, Sandulache VC, Simmons JC, Donovan DT, Ongkasuwan J. Causes and consequences of adult laryngotracheal stenosis. Laryngoscope. 2015;125:1137–43.
5. Shinn JR, Kimura KS, Campbell BR, et al. Incidence and outcomes of acute laryngeal injury after prolonged mechanical ventilation. Crit Care Med. 2019;47:1699–706.
6. Halum SL, Ting JY, Plowman EK, et al. A multi-institutional analysis of tracheotomy complications. Laryngoscope. 2012;122:38–45.
7. Carpenter DJ, Hamdi OA, Finberg AM, Daniero JJ. Laryngotracheal stenosis: mechanistic review. Head Neck. 2022;44(8):1948–60.
8. Namba DR, Ma G, Samad I, Ding D, Pandian V, Powell JD, Horton MR, Hillel AT. Rapamycin inhibits human laryngotracheal stenosis-derived fibroblast proliferation, metabolism, and function in vitro. Otolaryngol Head Neck Surg. 2015;152:881–8.
9. Ma G, Samad I, Motz K, Yin LX, Duvvuri MV, Ding D, Namba DR, Elisseeff JH, Horton MR, Hillel AT. Metabolic variations in normal and fibrotic human laryngotracheal-derived fibroblasts: a Warburg-like effect. Laryngoscope. 2017;127:E107–13.
10. Motz K, Samad I, Yin LX, Murphy MK, Duvvuri M, Ding D, Hillel AT. Interferon-γ treatment of human laryngotracheal stenosis-derived fibroblasts. JAMA Otolaryngol Head Neck Surg. 2017;143:1134–40.
11. Schoeff SS, Shi X, Young WG, Whited CW, Soni RS, Liu P, Ong IM, Dailey SH, Welham NV. Proteomic and genomic methylation signatures of idiopathic subglottic stenosis. Laryngoscope. 2021;131:E540–6.
12. Kemp WL, Burns DK, Brown TG. Inflammation and repair. In: Pathology: the big picture. New York: McGraw-Hill; 2008.
13. Bettinger DA, Yager DR, Diegelmann RF, Cohen IK. The effect of TGF-Beta on keloid fibroblast proliferation and collagen synthesis. Plast Reconstr Surg. 1996;98(5):827–33.
14. Franco RA Jr, Husain I, Reder L, Paddle P. Awake serial intralesional steroid injections without surgery as a novel targeted treatment for idiopathic subglottic stenosis. Laryngoscope. 2018;128(3):610–7.
15. Navani N, Costello D, Brown JM, Sandhu G, Janes SM, George J. A rare asthma mimic exposed by basic physiology. QJM. 2011;104:59–60.
16. Mokoka MC, Ullah K, Curran DR, O'Connor TM. Rare causes of persistent wheeze that mimic poorly controlled asthma. BMJ Case Rep. 2013;2013:bcr2013201100.
17. de Benedictis FM, de Benedictis D, Mirabile L, Pozzi M, Guerrieri A, Di Pillo S. Ground zero: not asthma at all. Pediatr Allergy Immunol. 2015;26:490–6.
18. Nouraei SAR, Nouraei SM, Patel A, Murphy K, Giussani DA, Koury EF, Brown JM, George PJ, Cummins AC, Sandhu GS. Diagnosis of laryngotracheal stenosis from routine pulmonary physiology using the expiratory disproportion index. Laryngoscope. 2013;123:3099–104.
19. Taha MS, Mostafa BE, Fahmy M, Ghaffar MKA, Ghany EA. Spiral CT virtual bronchoscopy with multiplanar reformatting in the evaluation of post-intubation tracheal stenosis: comparison between endoscopic, radiological and surgical findings. Eur Arch Otorrinolaringol. 2009;266:863–6.
20. Puchalski J, Musani AI. Tracheobronchial stenosis: causes and advances in management. Clin Chest Med. 2013;34:557–67.
21. Hseu AF, Benninger MS, Haffey TM, Lorenz R. Subglottic stenosis: a ten-year review of treatment outcomes. Laryngoscope. 2014;124(3):736–41.

22. Boyadjiev C, Popchristova E, Mazgalova J. Histomorphologic changes in keloids treated with Kenacort. J Trauma. 1995;38(2):299–302.
23. Cruz NI, Korchin L. Inhibition of human keloid fibroblast growth by isotretinoin and triamcinolone acetonide in vitro. Ann Plast Surg. 1994;33(4):401–5.
24. Reish RG, Eriksson E. Scar treatments: preclinical and clinical studies. J Am Coll Surg. 2008;206(4):719–30.
25. Hoffman MR, Coughlin AR, Dailey SH. Serial office-based steroid injections for treatment of idiopathic subglottic stenosis. Laryngoscope. 2017;127(11):2475–81.
26. Woliansky J, Phyland D, Paddle P. Systemic safety of serial intralesional steroid injection for subglottic stenosis. Laryngoscope. 2019;129(7):1634–9.
27. Pan DR, Rosow DE. Office-based corticosteroid injections as adjuvant therapy for subglottic stenosis. Laryngoscope Investig Otolaryngol. 2019;4(4):414–9.
28. Hoffman MR, Francis DO, Mai JP, Dailey SH. Office-based steroid injections for idiopathic subglottic stenosis: patient-reported outcomes, effect on stenosis, and side effects. Ann Otol Rhinol Laryngol. 2020;129(4):361–8.
29. Luke AS, Varelas EA, Kaplan S, Husain IA. Efficacy of office-based intralesional steroid injections in the management of subglottic stenosis: a systematic review. Ear Nose Throat J. 2023;102(6):372–8.
30. Schoeff S, Hoffman MR, Zhang Y, Yang Q, Dailey SH. Long-term follow-up of 64 patients with idiopathic subglottic stenosis: treatment pathways, outcomes, and impact of serial intralesional steroid injections. Ann Otol Rhinol Laryngol. 2023;132(11):1341–8.
31. Schuering JHC, van den Biesen SLG, van Benthem PPG, Sjögren EV, Langeveld APM. Office-based serial intralesional steroid injections in benign subglottic stenosis-first results. J Voice. 2024;S0892–1997(24)00416-8. https://doi.org/10.1016/j.jvoice.2024.11.036. Epub ahead of print. PMID: 39658425.

13 Complications and Adverse Effects Following Laryngeal Steroid Injections

With the growing literature on the use of intralesional steroid injection (ILSI) for the management of laryngeal disorders, there has been an increase in the number of complications. The most commonly reported are vocal fold submucosal hematoma and white plaque formation at the site of injection.

In a study of 126 patients who underwent ILSI for various vocal fold pathologies; Wang et al. reported hematoma and triamcinolone deposits in 27% and 4% of the cases, respectively [1]. In another study that included 24 patients with vocal fold polyps treated with triamcinolone acetonide injections (40 mg/ml), Hsu et al. reported a case of minor bleeding that resolved spontaneously [2]. Lee et al. described white plaque formation in 2 out of 80 patients with vocal fold nodules treated with ILSI. The plaque resolved spontaneously 4–8 weeks after treatment [3].

Another rare and feared complication of ILSI is vocal fold atrophy. Despite being diligent during an injection, inadvertent dissipation of glucocorticoid into the deep structures of the vocal folds may occur. This may lead to atrophy of the thyroarytenoid muscle, vocal ligament and or epithelial lining.

In 2011, Lee et al. reported 4 cases of mild vocal fold atrophy following ILSI for vocal fold nodules. Their study group consisted of 80 patients who were injected with a mean of 0.2 ml of triamcinolone acetonide suspension (40 mg/ml) into each vocal fold [3].

In 2014, Wang et al. reported vocal fold atrophy following ILSI in 1% of their study group, which consisted of 126 patients. The vocal fold atrophy resolved 4–8 weeks after treatment [1].

In 2016, Shi et al. reported two cases of vocal fold atrophy following serial vocal fold injections of steroids. The first patient was a case of vocal fold fibrosis post-radiation therapy who was treated with six corticoid injections (0.1 ml of dexamethasone/10 mg/ml) weekly. Although vocal fold injections were submucosal, the patient experienced worsening of his voice quality 1 week after the sixth injection. On laryngeal examination, there was atrophy of the injected vocal fold with incomplete closure of the vocal folds during phonation. The injections were stopped, and

A. L. Hamdan, *Atlas of Office-based Laryngeal Steroid Injection*,
https://doi.org/10.1007/978-3-032-05235-3_13

vocal fold atrophy resolved. The second patient was a case of Raynaud's phenomenon, esophageal dysmotility, sclerodactyly, and telangiectasia (CREST syndrome), who presented with a rough voice and increase phonatory effort. On laryngeal examination, she had decreased pliability of the vocal fold cover due to her primary disease. The patient was treated weekly with vocal fold steroid injections using dexamethasone (10 mg/ml). The treatment led to improvement in vocal fold stiffness initially; however, after the fifth injection, the patient had deterioration in her voice qualityHer voice became breathy, and laryngeal examination showed bilateral vocal fold atrophy, which improved after cessation of treatment [4].

These clinical cases are in agreement with animal studies documenting morphologic changes in muscle mass following repeated steroid injections. Hee-Jin et al. conducted a study examining histologic changes in the vocal folds of rabbits injected with triamcinolone and noted a significant degree of muscle atrophy that varied with the concentration of drug used across the three subgroups. The atrophy was observed at 4 weeks and recovered afterwards. Epithelial thinning was also observed at 2 weeks and lasted for 12 weeks [5]. The pathophysiology of thyroarytenoid muscle atrophy following steroid injection remains a subject of investigation.

Many mechanisms have been proposed, including alteration in myostatin expression—a master regulator of skeletal muscle mass that acts via a glucocorticoid receptor-mediated pathway [6]. Another suggested mechanism is the upregulation of Atrogin-1 and Muscle Ring Finger (MuRF-1), which enhance muscle proteolysis [7].

Gartling et al. conducted a pilot study on the impact of dexamethasone injection (40 microliters of 10 mg/ml dexamethasone) on thyroarytenoid-derived myoblasts isolated from Sprague-Dawley rats that were injected with 1 μM dexamethasone for 1 day, noting an increase in MuRF-1 gene expression. On the other hand, there was no increase in the TA MuRF-1 and Atrogin-1 expression, nor a decrease in the cross-sectional area of the TA muscles in thyroarytenoid muscle of New Zealand White rabbits that were sacrificed 7 days following dexamethasone injections [8].

Other less frequently reported complications of vocal fold steroid injections include narrowing of the airway secondary to over-injection and aspiration pneumonia because of anesthesia-induced impaired sensation in the larynx and pharynx [9]. Otolaryngologists should be aware of these rare complications and instruct the patient about them despite their rarity.

References

1. Wang CT, Lai MS, Hsiao TY. Comprehensive outcome researches of intralesional steroid injection on benign vocal fold lesions. J Voice. 2015;29(5):578–87.
2. Hsu YB, Lan MC, Chang SY. Percutaneous corticosteroid injection for vocal fold polyp. Arch Otolaryngol Head Neck Surg. 2009;135(8):776–80.
3. Lee S-H, Yeo J-O, Choi J-I, Jin H-J, Kim J-P, Woo S-H, Jin S-M. Local steroid injection via the cricothyroid membrane in patients with a vocal nodule. Arch Otolaryngol Head Neck Surg. 2011;137(10):1011–6.

4. Shi LL, Giraldez-Rodriguez LA, Johns MM III. The risk of vocal fold atrophy after serial corticosteroid injections of the vocal fold. J Voice. 2016;30(6):762–e11.
5. Jin HJ, Lee SH, Lee SU, Lee HS, Jin SM, Kim DH, Chae SW, Sohn JH. Morphological and histological changes of rabbit vocal fold after steroid injection. Otolaryngol Head Neck Surg. 2013;149(2):277–83.
6. Ma K, Mallidis C, Bhasin S, Mahabadi V, Artaza J, Gonzalez-Cadavid N, Arias J, Salehian B. Glucocorticoid-induced skeletal muscle atrophy is associated with upregulation of myostatin gene expression. Am J Physiol Endocrinol Metab. 2003;285(2):E363–71.
7. Langendorf EK, Rommens PM, Drees P, Mattyasovszky SG, Ritz U. Detecting the effects of the glucocorticoid dexamethasone on primary human skeletal muscle cells—differences to the murine cell line. Int J Mol Sci. 2020;21(7):2497.
8. Gartling G, Nakamura R, Sayce L, Zimmerman Z, Slater A, Wilson A, Bing R, Branski RC, Rousseau B. Acute in vitro and in vivo effects of dexamethasone in the vocal folds: a pilot study. Laryngoscope. 2023;133(9):2264–70.
9. Mallur PS, Rosen CA. Office-based laryngeal injections. Otolaryngol Clin N Am. 2013;46(1):85–100.

14 Conclusion

Glucocorticoid injections are frequently used to treat acute and chronic laryngeal inflammatory disorders. With the advances in technology and the introduction of a flexible endoscope with a working channel, laryngeal steroid injections are now easily performed in an office setting under local anesthesia. Their span of application has expanded to include the treatment of laryngeal scarring, infectious diseases, autoimmune disorders, and many exudative lesions of the lamina propria. Intralesional steroid injection (ILSI) has became an effective alternative to microlaryngeal surgery in the management of many voice disorders. If successfully performed, ILSI may obviate the need for surgical intervention in the operating room—thus sparing the patient the risks of general anesthesia and the morbidity of suspension microlaryngoscopy. In patients with vocal fold fibrosis, scars, and benign lesions of the vocal folds, the injection is usually made in the superficial layer of the lamina propria. The corticosteroid solution is typically injected into Reinke's space—and a bleb formation following the injection is considered by many laryngologists as a sign of a good injection. In many instances, more than one injection is needed to accomplish the desired effect.

The purpose of ILSI is to deliver a high drug concentration—while averting the adverse events of systemic therapy. The effect is mediated mostly by suppressing inflammatory markers such as interleukin-6 and tumor necrosis factor-alpha, among other factors. In patients with benign lesions of the vocal folds, ILSI can lead to partial or complete disease regression in the majority of cases. In patients with vocal fold cysts, disease regression following office-based intralesional steroid injection (ILSI) is also partially attributed to drainage of the cyst by the injecting needle during injection. When injected into a vocal fold scar, glucocorticoids many lead to improvement in voice quality and enhancement in vocal fold malleability by remodeling the lamina propria extracellular matrix.

Although laryngeal steroid injections are effective in the treatment of many laryngeal disorders, it is important to note that the success of these injections is contingent on many factors, such as patient selection, patient compliance, and the

A. L. Hamdan, *Atlas of Office-based Laryngeal Steroid Injection*, https://doi.org/10.1007/978-3-032-05235-3_14

approach used for the injection. Different approaches have been described in the literature. These include the peroral approach, the transnasal approach, and the percutaneous approach. This latter can be performed via the thyrohyoid membrane, thyroid cartilage, and the cricothyroid membrane. Choosing the appropriate approach for each patient might be a challenge. Patient-related factors—such as the anatomy of the neck and upper airway and the degree of gag reflex—warrant consideration. The success of ILSI is also contingent on the diligent application of local anesthetic to the larynx and pharynx—which remains the most crucial determinant for the completion of the procedure.

Complications following vocal fold steroid injection are rare. These include vocal fold hematoma, white plaque deposition, and vocal fold atrophy. These adverse events are invariably reversible with no long-term sequel. Patient counselling and reassurance are of paramount importance.

Index

A. L. Hamdan, *Atlas of Office-based Laryngeal Steroid Injection*,
https://doi.org/10.1007/978-3-032-05235-3

MIX
Papier aus verantwortungsvollen Quellen
Paper from responsible sources
FSC® C105338
FSC
www.fsc.org

If you have any concerns about our products,
you can contact us on
ProductSafety@springernature.com

In case Publisher is established outside the EU,
the EU authorized representative is:
Springer Nature Customer Service Center GmbH
Europaplatz 3, 69115 Heidelberg, Germany

Printed by Libri Plureos GmbH
in Hamburg, Germany